The Systematic Mistreatment of Children in the Foster Care System
Through the Cracks

The Haworth Press
Maltreatment, Trauma, and Interpersonal Aggression
Robert A. Geffner
Senior Editor

The Systematic Mistreatment of Children in the Foster Care System
Through the Cracks

Lois A. Weinberg

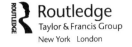

Routledge
Taylor & Francis Group
New York   London

For more information on this book or to order, visit
http://www.haworthpress.com/store/product.asp?sku=5136

or call 1-800-HAWORTH (800-429-6784) in the United States and Canada
or (607) 722-5857 outside the United States and Canada

or contact orders@HaworthPress.com

Published by

The Haworth Press, Taylor & Francis Group, 270 Madison Avenue, New York, NY 10016.

PUBLISHER'S NOTE
The development, preparation, and publication of this work has been undertaken with great care. However, the Publisher, employees, editors, and agents of The Haworth Press are not responsible for any errors contained herein or for consequences that may ensue from use of materials or information contained in this work. The Haworth Press is committed to the dissemination of ideas and information according to the highest standards of intellectual freedom and the free exchange of ideas. Statements made and opinions expressed in this publication do not necessarily reflect the views of the Publisher, Directors, management, or staff of The Haworth Press or an endorsement by them.

PUBLISHER'S NOTE

Identities and circumstances of individuals discussed in this book have been changed to protect confidentiality.

Excerpts from *Siblings in Out-of-Home Care: An Overview* reprinted by permission, © 2003 Casey Family Programs.

Library of Congress Cataloging-in-Publication Data

Weinberg, Lois A.
    The systematic mistreatment of children in the foster care system : through the cracks / Lois A Weinberg.
        p. cm.
    Includes bibliographical references.
    ISBN: 978-0-7890-2392-6 (hard)
    ISBN: 978-0-7890-2393-3 (soft)
    1. Foster children—United States. 2. Foster home care—United States. 3. Abused children—Services for—United States. 4. Child welfare—United States. I. Title.
HV875.55.W45 2007
362.73'30973—dc22
                                                                                    2007011205

To the memory of my parents, Etta and Arnold, who provided the type of safe, secure, and validating environment that was not available to the children described in this book.

ABOUT THE AUTHOR

Lois A. Weinberg, PhD, is an Associate Professor in the Division of Special Education and Counseling at California State University in Los Angeles, where she coordinates the CSULA-UCLA joint doctoral program in special education. She joined the faculty at CSULA in 2002 in the Mild to Moderate Disabilities Program. Prior to coming to CSULA, Dr. Weinberg was the Education Specialist at a nonprofit law office serving poor and low-income individuals with disabilities, where she provided advocacy for students in special education proceedings with a focus on children in the foster care system. She was also a Lecturer at the UCLA Graduate School of Education and Information Studies.

Dr. Weinberg co-directed the Education Initiative Project, a collaborative project in Los Angeles County designed to reduce educational barriers for foster children. With a grant from the Stuart Foundation, she works to help California counties improve the education of children in foster care. She has published numerous articles and made presentations across the country on the education of children in foster care, policy issues and services for children with emotional and behavioral disorders, and other policy issues in special education. Recent articles by Dr. Weinberg have appeared in *Child Abuse & Neglect, Children and Schools, Intervention in School & Clinic, Preventing School Failure,* and the *Journal of Education for Students Placed at Risk.*

CONTENTS

Preface

There are over 500,000 abused or neglected children in the United States who, on any given day, have been removed from the custody of their parents and placed in out-of-home placement—typically in a foster home, a small group home, or a large residential treatment facility (U.S. Department of Health and Human Services [U.S. DHSS], 2003). These are children for whom the state assumes responsibility for their safety, care, and overall well-being.

The Systematic Mistreatment of Children in the Foster Care System tells the stories of ten foster children[1] and the efforts by their advocates to bring about permanent places for them to live, appropriate schooling, and other services that were essential for their well-being. It highlights, through the use of actual case studies, the difficulty of placing and maintaining these children in appropriate living situations with supportive educational, mental health, and other services. Appropriate placement and services for these children typically requires the coordination and collaboration of several agencies—the juvenile court, child protective services (CPS), school districts, and departments of mental health (DMH), to name a few. Unfortunately, the structure of the multiagency system of care for many of these children does not work very well; it has "deep cracks," both within and between agencies, through which children in this system fall, sometimes over and over again.

These agencies were established or designated to provide services to either abused and neglected children or children with special needs because of a series of enlightened laws, passed over the last forty years. While these laws play an essential role in obtaining needed services for the children, they frequently are violated or are not sufficiently far reaching to overcome the tremendous problems in serving the needs of many children in the foster care system. *The Systematic*

The Systematic Mistreatment of Children in the Foster Care System
© 2007 by The Haworth Press, Taylor & Francis Group. All rights reserved.
doi:10.1300/5136_a

Mistreatment of Children in the Foster Care System shows how the various agencies responsible for children in the foster care system frequently fail to meet their legal obligations toward these children. The book also shows important avenues for addressing these failures and the outcomes they produce.

The book is based on a case study (Weinberg, 1997; Weinberg, Weinberg, & Shea, 1997) of the responses of educational, child protective services, and other agencies to efforts by legal advocates to secure services for a group of neglected children from diverse ethnic and cultural backgrounds. The detailed stories of these efforts for ten of the children form the basis for the cases presented in this book. The book focuses on the crucial need for changes in how we serve this vulnerable, culturally diverse population of children.

The Systematic Mistreatment of Children in the Foster Care System is divided into twelve chapters. The first two chapters provide an introduction to the child protective services system and the educational system in order to give readers the requisite background for understanding the cases of the children presented in the chapters that follow.

The next ten chapters consist of the case studies of the children. These chapters are categorized by a major issue presented in the case. Each of the chapters in these three sections includes:

- An introduction to the specific issue or issues presented in the chapter
- A case study of a child that illustrates and illuminates the issue(s)
- Subsections titled *Prevention* that discuss actions taken to prevent further child abuse or neglect for the child in the case study;
- Subsections titled *Intervention* that describe the specific interventions that occurred either to reduce the effects of the trauma the child in the case study had experienced or to provide needed educational or other services to maintain a child in a placement
- Subsections called *What Had Gone Wrong?* that describe the specific problems or legal violations that occurred in trying to obtain for the child in the case study appropriate and needed services
- Subsections titled *Advocacy Considerations* that describe why the advocates for the child used the strategies that they did to try

to overcome legal violations or to garner specific services or placements
- A conclusion delineating the effect of the advocacy endeavors for the child and the difficulties the case presented and
- A summary, highlighting the purpose of the chapter

Chapter 12 focuses on policy implications and provides directions for change so that fewer children in foster care will experience the problems described in the case studies.

The primary audience for *The Systematic Mistreatment of Children in the Foster Care System* includes professionals, academics, and undergraduate and graduate college and university students in the fields of social work, education, public policy, psychology, and law. Juvenile court attorneys, judges, and others involved in the representation or care (e.g., foster parents, residential treatment administrators and staff) of abused and neglected children should find the cases of the children and the struggles to procure appropriate services for them familiar. Policymakers, hopefully, will find this book useful in evaluating the types of policy decisions at the federal, state, and local levels that are needed to better provide for this population of children. Ideally, there will be interest in the book from the general reading public concerned about society's vulnerable, at-risk children.

The details of the children's lives, the interventions made on their behalf by those of us at Advocacy Services,[2] and the responses to these interventions fill most of the chapters of this book. I have tried to present each child as an individual so that the reader comes to know the struggles of each and, in some cases, the resilience against tremendous odds. I also have tried to present the interventions made by the staff at Advocacy Services in a way that the reader comes to understand the types of service needs the children have, the various agencies responsible for meeting these needs, and the problems encountered by us in trying to get their needs met. I have once again, as part of writing this book, returned to the children's case records so that the details presented here are as accurate as possible while, at the same time, writing in such a way as to protect their anonymity.

Acknowledgments

There are many people who helped me along the way making writing this book possible for me. Jeannie Oakes, professor of urban studies at UCLA, was the first to suggest that I write a book after hearing me describe the particular struggles of the children described here and our advocacy efforts on their behalf. Carl Weinberg, my husband and a professor emeritus at UCLA, was a constant and invaluable source of support and encouragement during my writing of the book. He read every chapter, some more than once, and suggested changes that helped to make this a better-written book than it would have been without his recommendations. Deborah Stipek, dean of the School of Education at Stanford, provided ongoing encouragement for me to seek out publishers and checked in with me on a regular basis to see how I was progressing in completing the manuscript.

This book would not have been possible without the hard work and committed advocacy of my colleagues at the law firm. Nancy Shea, senior attorney, appointed by the juvenile court to represent all of the children, always was clear that education was important for foster youth before others began to realize this obvious fact. She also knew that these young people needed a coordinated set of services to reach their potential and was extremely knowledgeable about how to bring this about. Nancy also requested and was granted permission from the presiding judge of the juvenile court for me to write about the children in this book, with the proviso that I did not reveal who they were. I believe I have maintained their confidentiality by not revealing their actual names, caretakers, schools, dates when incidents took place, or the locale where the children lived. I also have changed some of the facts of their lives to further protect their confidentiality. Any inaccuracies that exist in how I have described or analyzed the cases or in the advocacy solutions discussed are mine alone and should not be attributed to the law firm or any individual working there.

Pam Marx, staff attorney, joined the team after Nancy and I had started working on the children's cases, but was quick to discern what services they needed, stayed in close contact with the children and their caretakers, and was frequently quite creative in her solutions to their problems. Jim Preis, executive director of the law firm, believed strongly in the professional capabilities of those of us who provided advocacy for the children, gave us the latitude to use our judgment in advocating for them, but also provided an important sounding board and guidance when needed.

I always will be grateful to Bob Geffner, editor of The Haworth Press Maltreatment, Trauma, and Interpersonal Aggression book series, for recognizing the value of the children's stories and suggesting that The Haworth Press publish this book. I also credit him with recommending a structure for the stories of the children that I believe leads to a more thorough understanding of the work we did on their behalf and will help others to learn from our advocacy efforts. Terry S. Trepper, editor in chief of the Behavioral and Social Sciences book program at Haworth, provided critical feedback on a draft of the manuscript.

There are others at The Haworth Press whom I also would like to thank for their efforts in moving the manuscript forward to publication: Rebecca Browne, project manager, Mary Beth Madden, associate production editor, and Amy Rentner, senior production editor. I also am grateful for the thorough editing of the manuscript by Vidhya Jayaprakash, production manager, and her copyediting team at Newgen Imaging Systems.

Chapter 1

The Child Protective System

This chapter describes the general route by which children in the United States are removed from the custody of their parents because of abuse or neglect. While the specifics may differ to some extent depending on the particular state or county, the path itself is similar to that experienced by the almost 800,000 abused and neglected children each year across the country who are removed from their parent's custody (Adoption and Foster Care Analysis and Reporting System [AFCARS], 2006a; AFCARS, 2006b). The process described in this chapter serves as background to the cases of the ten children that are delineated in this book.

REPORTING ABUSE OR NEGLECT

The road for each of the children, which culminated in the child's removal from the custody of their parents, started with a call to a child protective services (CPS) agency with a report of suspicion of abuse or neglect. In Patty's case, for example, her father made the first call to CPS reporting that the sons of his ex-wife had molested her, leading to a short removal from the home when she was ten. Several months later, however, a family in the community who were providing childcare to her made the next report after Patty climbed on an adult male in the home and began rubbing against him sexually.

Sharon's sexual abuse, when she was five, was discovered by a member of a hospital pediatric-child-abuse project. These pediatric practitioners were legally required, as mandated reporters, to report

The Systematic Mistreatment of Children in the Foster Care System
© 2007 by The Haworth Press, Taylor & Francis Group. All rights reserved.
doi:10.1300/5136_01

their discovery to CPS, which they did. A teacher, also a mandated reporter, reported suspected physical abuse of Silvia and Carlos' older sister. This report triggered an investigation by CPS.

Until the mid-1960s, no state in the United States had a law that required the reporting of child abuse (Besharov, 1985). However, beginning in the mid-1960s and continuing through the 1970s all fifty states had passed new child maltreatment reporting laws (Faller, 1985). These state laws clarified the duty of professionals to report known or suspected child abuse or neglect. In 1974, the passage of the Child Abuse Prevention and Treatment Act (CAPTA) by the U.S. Congress set in motion a comprehensive system of child protection and helped ensure substantial uniformity among the reporting laws of the fifty states (see Exhibit 1.1).

All states now have mandatory reporting laws typically based on a reasonable suspicion or knowledge of current abuse or neglect (Child Welfare Information Gateway, 2005c). Professionals who fall under the reporting laws must, under threat of criminal or civil penalties, report known and suspected child abuse or neglect (Mason & Gambull, 1994). Mandatory reporters typically include physicians, nurses, teachers, daycare providers, law enforcement personnel, social workers, and other mental health professionals. In some states, everyone in the state has a duty to report any reasonable suspicion of child abuse or neglect, not just certain classes of professionals (Besharov, 1985; Child Welfare Information Gateway, 2005c). Many CPS agencies have established "hotlines" to make the reporting of child abuse or neglect a fairly simple and routine matter (Reed & Karpilow, 2002).

EXHIBIT 1.1.
Child Abuse Prevention and Treatment Act (CAPTA)

The passage of CAPTA, Public Law 93-247, in 1974 mandated that states establish child abuse reporting laws, define child abuse and neglect, describe the circumstances and conditions that obligate mandated reporters to report known or suspected child abuse, determine when juvenile/family courts can take custody of a child, and specify the forms of maltreatment that are criminally punishable. CAPTA has been amended and reauthorized several times since its inception.

INVESTIGATION

Once a report of abuse or neglect is made, CPS first determines through a screening process if there is sufficient evidence to warrant an in-person investigation (Reed & Karpilow, 2002). If so, CPS initiates an intake investigation to gather as much information about the alleged incident as quickly as possible. Depending on case circumstances, this investigation may take only a few hours or may take as long as a couple of months, (McCarthy, Marshall, Arganza, Deserley, & Milon, 2005; Weisz, 1995). However, staff shortages in CPS agencies limit the investigations (Besharov, 1983; Child Welfare League of America [CWLA], 2002a; Gunderson & Osborne, 2001) along with a lack of investigative technology, training, and resources (Lindsey, 2004).

The investigation of abuse and neglect claims typically consists of a CPS worker visiting the home to interview the child and parent (or other caregiver) and assess the home environment (Badeau & Gesiriech, 2003). CPS also interviews, usually by telephone, the person who made the child abuse or neglect report (Carroll & Haase, 1988). In Patty's case, the initial investigation by CPS led to her allegation that her father, as well as her former stepbrother, had molested her.

The purpose of the intake investigation is to determine whether a child's parent or caregiver has engaged in behavior that is prohibited by the abuse or neglect laws. If the investigation reveals substantial evidence of abuse or neglect, the CPS worker makes a determination as to the present risk to the child. The child is either left in the home, sometimes with protective services provided; or removed and placed with a relative; in a foster home; or in a temporary shelter. Anthony's first placement was in the county emergency shelter. Patty was initially placed in a foster home, while James, whose mother's drug-addiction led to her abusing and neglecting him, was placed with his grandmother. For Patty, this initial placement lasted for a very short time, with a great many placements following. James stayed with his grandmother for quite a while, until she was no longer able to care for him. He too then found himself being discharged from one living situation after another.

THE PETITION

When the CPS worker makes a determination that the child cannot be protected and remain safely in the home, even with supportive services provided, a petition must be filed by the agency requesting immediate custody of the child (Badeau & Gesiriech, 2003). For each of the children's cases described in this book, CPS filed such a petition.

The petition is the legal document by which the court gains jurisdiction over the child and parents. It lists the specific allegations of child abuse or neglect against the parents, which correspond to state law. A copy of the petition is served individually to each parent of the child as well as notice of subsequent court hearings. By law, removing a child from his or her parents' home should not occur without a court hearing, except in cases that constitute an emergency in terms of protecting the safety or health of the child. Nevertheless, in most cases, removal of the child from the parents' home occurs pending a preliminary hearing on the need to take immediate custody of the child (Pellman, 1996; Meddin & Hansen, 1985). For the cases of the children described in this book, the law requires CPS to file a petition within forty-eight hours of detaining the child, and a hearing takes place within seventy-two hours of detention (Pellman, 1996). Other states have similar timelines regarding filing petitions and holding hearings for children detained for abuse or neglect.

When the primary service delivered at this stage of the process is out-of-home placement, rather than in-home services that might avoid such placement, CPS may not be meeting its mandate of preplacement preventive services under the Adoption Assistance and Child Welfare Act (Meddin & Hansen, 1985). In addition, a high percentage of children who are at risk of out-of-home placement because of abuse or neglect may be able to remain at home if intensive, preventive services are provided to their families (Bower, 2003; Burchard, Burns, & Burchard, 2002). However, there is significantly more funding available to support foster and adoptive families than birth parents, making it difficult for CPS to provide prevention services to resolve crises before removing children from their parents (Reed & Karpilow, 2002). It is possible that John, for example, a child whose mother employed abusive punishment in an attempt to curb his hyperactive behavior, might have been able to remain in the home with his mother, if such intensive services had been available (see Exhibit 1.2).

THE COURT

It is important to realize that the court involved in child protection cases, depending on the state, is the juvenile, family, or sometimes the probate court, rather than the criminal court (Schweitzer & Larsen, 2005). In some jurisdictions, the juvenile court is divided into the delinquency court and the dependency court. When this division exists, it is the juvenile dependency court that has jurisdiction over cases of child abuse or neglect. The purpose of the juvenile dependency court is to protect the child if it is determined that he or she is abused or neglected (Weisz, 1995).

The distinguishing feature of the juvenile dependency court is that it acts as an arbiter of personal liberty and must assure that the rights of parents, children, and society are protected (Besharov, 1985). The personal rights at stake for both parents and children, when there are questions of abuse or neglect, have been recognized as fundamentally important constitutional rights (*Meyer v. Nebraska,* 1963; *Pierce v. Society of Sisters,* 1925; *Griswold v. Connecticut,* 1965). These rights are both those of parents to the care and custody of their children, and those of children to live with their parents without governmental interference. The juvenile or family court only may infringe upon these rights after due process of law.

EXHIBIT 1.2.
Adoption Assistance and Child Welfare Act

In 1980, Public Law 96-272 created a categorical funding stream for out-of-home care of foster youth to support the goal of protecting children, but also established a preference to maintain and reunify families. This Act requires reasonable efforts to prevent unnecessary out-of-home placements, requires consideration of relatives as the placement of preference, establishes a process to safely reunify children with their families when possible, and authorizes assistance payments to families who adopt children with special needs.

The court must decide whether the circumstances in the case justify coercive, authoritative state intervention on behalf of the child.

Legal Representation and Court-Appointed Advocates

In order for a state to receive funds under CAPTA, the state must establish procedures requiring the appointment of a *guardian ad litem* in every case involving an abused or neglected child that results in a judicial proceeding. A guardian ad litem may be either an attorney or a court-appointed-special advocate (CASA) who is appointed to represent the child. According to CAPTA, the guardian ad litem is to obtain a firsthand, clear understanding of the child's situation and needs and to make recommendations to the court concerning the best interests of the child. There may be a conflict when an attorney is the guardian ad litem, however, since an attorney's duty is to achieve the child's legal goals, taking into account the child's age and development, which, at times, may be at odds with what is in the child's best interests (Schweitzer & Larsen, 2005) (see Exhibit 1.3).

For the children described in this book, each had representation by an attorney appointed by the juvenile court. In addition, the child's parents were appointed an attorney and the CPS agency had attorney representation. David, in addition to attorney representation, also had a CASA assigned to his case. CASAs are trained volunteers who attend court hearings, help to ensure court-ordered services are provided to the child, monitor services, report to the court, and provide continuity and a stable presence in the child's life. In the county where David lived, there are not enough CASAs available and, therefore,

---

EXHIBIT 1.3.
Guardian Ad Litem

Ad litem in Latin means "for the purpose of the legal action only." A guardian ad litem is a guardian appointed by a court in a particular legal matter to protect the interests of a minor or person deemed incompetent. State law and local court rules govern the appointment of guardian ad litems. Typically, the court may appoint either a lawyer or a court-appointed special advocate to serve as guardian ad litem in juvenile and family court matters.

they are assigned only to a small number of cases of foster youth with special needs.

COURT PROCEEDINGS

Detention/Arraignment Hearings

The first court hearing for a child may last only long enough for the judge (or other judicial officer[1]) to hear sufficient evidence in support of the allegations in the petition to warrant keeping the child out of the home until the adjudication hearing. The detention hearing involves decisions about detaining a child, whether reasonable efforts were expended in trying to prevent out-of-home placement, and with whom the child will remain temporarily. Once these decisions are made, the arraignment may follow. It is at the arraignment hearing where the parents' attorney typically will enter a general denial to the allegations of abuse or neglect against the parents that appear in the petition (Pellman, 1996).

Adjudication Hearing

Before the full hearing on the issues in the case, which is called an adjudication, the parties may use a pretrial negotiation or mediation process to try to reach agreement on all or part of the issues. For the cases that do not settle, a full hearing on the issues takes place. A judge hears evidence as to whether the allegations in the petition are true. The respective attorneys for the parents, the child, and CPS may present evidence at the hearing through the sworn testimony of witnesses and the acceptance of documents and other material into evidence. They also may cross-examine witnesses. The purpose of the testimony and other evidence is to support or refute the allegations of abuse or neglect in the petition. The burden of proving child abuse or neglect is on CPS (Pellman, 1996). After all the evidence is heard, the judge will make a finding as to whether the allegations of abuse or neglect in the petition were upheld, and if so, where the child is to remain until the disposition hearing.

The federal statute, CAPTA (2003), defines child abuse and neglect as the physical or mental injury, sexual abuse, negligent treatment, or maltreatment of a child under the age of 18 by a person who is responsible for the child's welfare under circumstances which indicate that the child's health or welfare is harmed or threatened (see Exhibit 1.4).

Physical Abuse

All U.S. states and territories provide a definition of physical abuse (Child Welfare Information Gateway, 2005b). The term generally is defined as serious physical harm inflicted nonaccidentally by the child's parent or guardian (Child Welfare Information Gateway, 2005a). CPS initially removed Sharon from the custody of her mother because of nonaccidentally inflicted physical abuse. John, James, and Robert also were removed from their parent's custody because of physical abuse.

Neglect

Neglect also is addressed in the statutes of all U.S. states and territories, either as a separate definition or as a part of abuse (Child Welfare Information Gateway, 2005b). Neglect is serious physical harm or illness as the result of the failure to provide adequate food, shelter, or medical treatment (Child Welfare Information Gateway, 2005a). Some states also include the failure of a child's parent or guardian to adequately supervise or protect the child. Anthony's father, who had a developmental disability, had failed to care for him or provide adequate food. Silvia, Carlos, and James all suffered from parental neglect because of their parents' substance abuse. Patty's father had

---

EXHIBIT 1.4.
Definition of Abuse and Neglect

The physical or mental injury, sexual abuse, negligent treatment, or maltreatment of a child under the age of 18 by a person who is responsible for the child's welfare under circumstances which indicate that the child's health or welfare is harmed or threatened thereby. (CAPTA, 2003, §5106(g))

failed to adequately supervise her and obtain necessary counseling to correct her inappropriate sexual behavior.

Emotional Abuse

Most states and territories include emotional maltreatment as part of their definitions of abuse or neglect (Child Welfare Information Gateway, 2005b). This type of abuse involves serious emotional damage, as a result of the conduct of the parent or guardian. None of the ten children were removed from their parents' custody for emotional damage, although the emotional damage many of the children suffered is quite apparent from their stories.

Sexual Abuse

All states include sexual abuse in their definitions (Child Welfare Information Gateway, 2005b). Some states refer to sexual abuse in general terms while others identify specific acts (Child Welfare Information Gateway, 2005b). The second time CPS removed Sharon from her mother's custody was because of sexual abuse. Her mother had failed to adequately protect her from sexual abuse, most likely, by her uncle.

Abandonment

Many states provide definitions of child abandonment (Child Welfare Information Gateway, 2005b). Abandonment occurs when the child has been left without any provision for support, the parent has failed to maintain contact with the child, or whereabouts of the parent is unknown (Child Welfare Information Gateway, 2005a). David's mother abandoned him, as did Debra's caregiver.

Disposition Hearing

After the adjudication, a disposition hearing is scheduled. The primary purpose of the disposition hearing is to determine who should have legal custody of the child, where the child will live, and what services the child and family will receive based on what is thought to be in the best interest of the child (Schweitzer & Larsen, 2005; Weisz,

1996). The Adoption and Safe Families Act (ASFA) (1997) requires a case plan be developed that stresses the child's health and safety as paramount concern. The case plan includes: the permanent long-term placement goal for the child (e.g., reunification with the parents, permanent out-of-home placement, adoption); the services to be provided to attain that goal; the parents' responsibilities if reunification with the child is the eventual goal; the child's responsibilities, if any; a description of the child's placement; and arrangements for maintaining contact between the child and parents (see Exhibit 1.5).

There are two general categories of placement options—home of parent and suitable placement—when the court takes jurisdiction of the child and the child becomes a dependent (i.e., the child's custody and care become the responsibility of CPS).

Home of Parent

The child is returned to the parents' home but the court still has jurisdiction. John, Robert, and James, for short periods, were returned to their parents' homes; but these placements were never successful for very long. Had certain supportive services been put in place, particularly in John's case, being placed in his mother's home might have been successful.

EXHIBIT 1.5.
Adoption and Safe Families Act (ASFA)

ASFA, PL 105-89, made the most significant changes to the child welfare provisions since they were established in their modern form in 1980. The Act emphasizes child safety over keeping families together and provides financial incentives to states to promote permanency planning and adoption. It establishes expedited timelines for determining whether children who enter foster care can be moved into permanent homes promptly. Permanency hearings must be held for children no later than twelve months after they enter foster care (six months earlier than under prior law). Termination of parental rights proceedings are to be initiated for children who have been under the responsibility of the state for fifteen out of the most recent twenty-two months, unless certain exceptions apply.

Suitable Placement

The child is placed outside of the family residence typically in the home of a relative, a foster home, or a group home. In some jurisdictions, there are temporary-emergency shelters or state hospitals for youngsters with severe mental disabilities.

The "home of relative" option, also known as kinship care, is placement with a member of a child's extended family who may be entitled to some funding to help care for the child (*Miller v. Yoakim,* 1979). CPS placed James with his grandmother until she became too frail to care for him. He also lived briefly with his aunt. Carlos' placement was with an aunt and uncle for a very short period.

A "foster home" refers to a placement with a family or a single adult (not related to the child) whose home is licensed by the state to house a certain number of foster children for whom the foster parent receives funding. There are specialized foster homes for which foster parents receive a higher rate of funding to care for children with physical or mental health needs. Silvia was placed in a foster home, as were Carlos, Debra, and Sharon. Debra's foster home received a higher rate of funding for her care because of her mental retardation. Silvia was the only one of the children who remained with the same foster family.

"Group Homes" are either community homes or large-scale facilities, which contain between six and several hundred children and are staffed by twenty-four-hour childcare workers. Children who are hard-to-place because of emotional or behavioral problems are more likely to be placed in group homes (Pellman, 1996). Seven of the children spent time in six-bed group homes, while eight were placed for periods in larger residential facilities.

In the case of the children described in this book, "emergency shelter" refers to a county placement that housed between 200 and 250 youngsters between the ages of birth and nineteen years and was intended as a temporary placement of fifteen to thirty days (Pellman, 1996). Seven children were placed in the county emergency shelter, some for many months to over a year.

"State hospitals" are for those with mental illness or developmental disabilities and for whom community placements are not appropriate. None of the ten children were placed in a state hospital. Advocacy efforts were successful in keeping Patty and Sharon, out of the state hospital (see Exhibit 1.6).

EXHIBIT 1.6.
Placement Options

Home of Parent—Child is returned to the parents' home but the court still has jurisdiction.
Suitable Placement—Child is placed outside of the family residence in the home of a relative, a foster family, or in group care.

Placement Considerations

ASFA (1997) requires that a child's health and safety must be paramount when decisions are made about the initial removal of a child from his or her home, the reunification with a child's parents, and the care a child receives while in foster care or in an adoptive family. Other factors a court may take into account when making a decision about a child's placement include: extended family support; willingness of the parent to receive in-home services; willingness of the parent to participate in court-ordered services such as counseling or drug rehabilitation programs and testing; age of the child; medical and psychological history of the child; substance abuse history of the parents; and juvenile court referrals of the parents (Weisz, 1996).

Weisz (1996) argues that the CPS system is structured in such a way as to focus primarily on short-term intervention. However, as with the cases described in this book, many maltreating families experience chronic, and multiple, crises and require ongoing support and services, often until the children become adults. If children are to remain in the homes of these families rather than be placed in out-of home placement, communities must accept responsibility for providing comprehensive services to families on a long-term basis (CWLA, 2002b; Weisz, 1996). Unfortunately, because of high caseloads, CPS workers are not available to reach out and work intensively with families in the context of their homes (Weisz, 1996). They may not focus, for example, on such concrete family problems and stresses as inadequate housing and unemployment as factors appropriate for their intervention. Some of these factors were relevant in John's need for an out-of-home placement.

Review Hearings

AFSA (1997) requires periodic review hearings following the disposition of the case to ensure that a permanent placement is found for the child without unnecessary delay. According to AFSA, reviews must be held six months after the disposition and permanency decisions now must be made no longer than twelve months after the initial out-of-home placement. For the children described in this book, review hearings were required every six months; however, finding permanent placements remained elusive for most of them. For the children described in this book who were placed at the county emergency shelter, review hearings were required every fifteen days.

The juvenile dependency court retains ultimate responsibility for the well-being of children under its jurisdiction. The review hearings provide an avenue for ongoing court review of the case treatment or permanency plan. CPS must give an account to the court of what services have been provided and what progress the family has made. The parents must show what progress they have made in correcting the problems that brought their child to the attention of the court and their adherence with the case plan (Schweitzer & Larsen, 2005). The attorneys representing the children present to the court at these hearings the children's desires and needs. CASAs report on what is in the best interests of the child. Dependency court judges also may hear from the children themselves. The case plans may be clarified or revised at the review hearings based on the actions of the parents, the CPS agency, and the needs of the child. Visitation of the child by the parents may be required along with required treatment programs and services. For the ten children, placement decisions were sometimes changed at these hearings as well as court orders made for various services. For example, James' mother was required to enroll in a drug rehabilitation program and Anthony's mother was required to attend psychiatric counseling. If parents do not follow the requirements of the case plan, their rights as parents may ultimately be terminated.

ROLE OF THE CHILD'S ATTORNEY

The previous section delineated the process by which the juvenile court becomes involved in the lives of children who are removed from their parents' custody because of abuse or neglect. This section focuses on the role of the child's attorney. For those states where attorneys are appointed to represent children in dependency proceedings, they may oversee the child's case from the time they are appointed until the court terminates its jurisdiction of the child. Frequently, their role in providing adequate representation for the child is far more than simply appearing at hearings, making motions, and filing briefs. Successful advocacy, as exhibited by the stories of the children in this book, requires regular interaction with the CPS worker and other agency personnel who provide services to the child, such as mental health professionals, foster parents, group home staff, teachers, and others. Since the CPS agency has primary responsibility for the decisions regarding protection and placement of the child, subject to court approval, it is important for those representing the child to have a working relationship with the CPS worker in order to influence decisions affecting the child. Such a working relationship, for example, was crucial in keeping Sharon out of the delinquency system. These decisions can include developing the case plan for the child, monitoring whether all aspects of the case plan are carried out, recommending changes in the case plan when needed, and monitoring the quality of care and services the child receives. For many court-appointed attorneys who represent children in a juvenile court, the reality of their enormous caseloads precludes the kind of out-of-court advocacy described here.

CRACKS IN THE CHILD PROTECTIVE SYSTEM

There has been considerable criticism in recent years about the negative impact on children of a child protective system that ostensibly is set up to protect them. Criticisms are wide-ranging and focus on many different aspects of the system that cause unintentional mistreatment by those agencies whose job is to protect abused or neglected children. This mistreatment has been attributed to such factors as: a shortage of social workers; high caseloads; lack of meaningful contact with children and families (Reed & Karpilow, 2002); caseworkers left to make too many decisions alone, without adequate training, supervision, or guidelines (National Council of Juvenile and Family Court Judges [NCJFCJ], 1986); the lack of immediate and effective treatment and coordinated planning and resources, (NCJFCJ, 1986; Soler & Schauffer, 1990); and an inadequate number of available resources (Janko, 1994; Jellinek, Murphy, Poitrast, Gwinn, Bishop, & Goshko, 1992; Wald & Wolverton, 1990).

In addition, CPS has a differential effect on different cultural and racial groups. In particular, African-American children are more likely to enter the CPS system at younger ages, be placed in foster care, spend more time in the system, and experience multiple foster care placements (U.S. DHHS Bureau, 1997). While abused and neglected children in general face daunting problems as they negotiate the system of multiple agencies responsible for their care, these problems multiply considerably for abused and neglected children with disabilities, as is seen in the stories of the children in this book. There is currently a woeful lack of sufficiently trained foster parents and specialized foster homes (NCJFCJ, 1986). Inadequate screenings and a lack of coordination between services frequently result in the failure to provide appropriate services (NCJFCJ, 1986). Also, there is an insufficient number of quality group homes and residential treatment programs as well as quality mental health and educational services (Bauer, 1993; Howing & Wodarski, 1992; Knitzer, 1982). For the children whose stories are told in this book, there are cracks in each of the various agencies set up for their protection, education, and care. And these cracks widen considerably when malfunctioning agencies must collaborate in the overall interest of the child. Hopefully, in the cases to follow, many of those cracks will be exposed and some solutions suggested such that child welfare policy and the subsequent treatment of abused and neglected children can be improved.

SUMMARY

The purpose of this chapter was to describe the process by which children in the United States are removed from the custody of their parents because of abuse or neglect. The process described includes the reporting of suspected abuse or neglect, the investigation of abuse and neglect allegations by CPS, and the role of the juvenile court and procedures when CPS determines that a child cannot remain safely in the home of their parents. The chapter delineates the different types of juvenile court hearings—detention/arraignment, adjudication, disposition, and periodic review—along with the possible categories of abuse and neglect allegations. In addition, there is a description of the various types of placement options typically available when children are placed in out-of home care by the juvenile court. Furthermore, there are criticisms against a child protective system that has as its purpose to protect children who have been abused or neglected but frequently affects these children in very negative ways. The chapter illuminates the process of removing children from their parents' homes and custody with examples of the children whose cases are described in more detail in other chapters of the book.

Chapter 2

The Educational System

All the children described in this book had learning or emotional problems that affected their educational performance and functioning in school. In some cases, there were disabilities with known causes, such as with Patty who had a traumatic brain injury from an automobile accident; in most cases, however, the causes of their learning and other school problems were not known, although, prenatal exposure to alcohol or drugs, early neglect, physical or sexual abuse, and genetic predisposition were suspected. In addition, their lives in the foster care system—lack of home or school stability, excessive time out of school, failure to receive appropriate schooling, mental health, or other services—exacerbated whatever problems they had when they entered the system.

All of the children began receiving special education services to address their educational needs; although some, such as Silvia, Carlos, John, and, perhaps, James might not have had "disabilities" if they had had different life situations. They might then have been able to progress in school simply with general education options.

Obtaining the appropriate special education services for the children, more often than not, was frequently quite difficult, even with skilled advocacy. The process of navigating the special education system, from the initial referral stage to placement in a classroom with special instruction and services many times is daunting for children whose parents are dedicated advocates for them. For children who do not live with their parents, who are in out-of-home placement, and who suffer the consequences of abuse or neglect, the special education system often is extremely difficult to negotiate (Choice et al., 2001; Weinberg, 1997).

The Systematic Mistreatment of Children in the Foster Care System
© 2007 by The Haworth Press, Taylor & Francis Group. All rights reserved.
doi:10.1300/5136_02

Some children in foster care end up in special education programs when, in fact, they do not have disabilities. This may happen because they are placed in a group home that has an on-grounds special education school, and all the children in the home then become eligible for these special education services. There also are times when children enter foster care emotionally distraught due to the upheaval in their lives related to the removal from their parents' home and placement in foster care. Their behavior during this time may be misinterpreted as emotional disturbance, thus qualifying them for special education.

FOSTER CHILDREN AND DISABILITIES

Special education is a program, mandated by a federal law titled the Individuals with Disabilities Education Act (IDEA) (2004), which was originally passed by the U.S. Congress in 1975 as the Education for All Handicapped Children Act. This law provides specially designed instruction and services to children with disabilities. Approximately 12 percent of students six to twenty-one years enrolled in public school have disabilities, thus entitling them to receive special education services (U.S. Department of Education, 2003; see Exhibit 2.1).

It is not known how many foster children nationwide receive special education services. Depending on the sample studied, the percentage of children in foster care receiving special education ranges somewhere between 30 and 50 percent (Berrick, Courtney, & Barth, 1993; Courtney, Terao, & Bost, 2004; Goerge, Voorhis, Grant, Casey, & Robinson, 1992; Hochstadt, Jaudes, Zimo, & Schachter, 1987; see Exhibit 2.2).

EXHIBIT 2.1.
Individual with Disabilities Education Act

A federal law that requires specially designed instruction and services in the least restrictive environment to eligible students with disabilities. (IDEA, 2004)

EXHIBIT 2.2.
Percentage of Students Receiving
Special Education Services

- 9 percent of elementary and secondary students receive special education services. (Hunt & Marshall, 2005)
- 30 percent to 52 percent of foster youth receive special education services. (Weinberg, Zetlin, & Shea, 2001)

It is not surprising that a higher percentage of children in foster care receive special education services than children in the general school-age population, since a large percentage of children in foster care are reported to have conditions that might make them eligible for these services. Bauer (1993) reported that 25 percent of children in foster care have disabilities. Richardson and her colleagues (1989) found that 40 percent of all children in out-of-home care are developmentally delayed. In a study by McIntyre and Keesler (1986), nearly half the population of children in foster care manifested evidence of psychological disorders. Courtney, Terao, and Bost (2004) found that 31 percent of foster youth in three midwestern states had one or more mental health or behavioral disorders. Studies from the U.S. General Accounting Office (1995) indicate that as many as 58 percent of children in foster care have serious health problems.

Abused and neglected children, when compared with nonmaltreated children, also have been shown to have a wide range of school indicators that may suggest the possibility of disabilities or simply indicate the difficult lives they have had, such as lower academic performance, poorer grades, higher grade retention, more disciplinary problems, and greater absenteeism. Eckenrode, Laird, and Doris (1993) found that abused and neglected children performed significantly lower on standardized achievement tests in reading and mathematics, earned lower grades in these subjects, were likely to repeat a grade, and had higher rates of disciplinary referrals. Kurtz and his colleagues (1993) found that children who had been physically abused and those who had been neglected had significantly lower verbal, mathematics, and overall achievement, as measured by standardized test scores, grades, teacher assessments, and grade retentions. Teachers and parents rated the children who experienced physical abuse as having more behavior problems than the nonmaltreated or neglected children. In a study by Leiter and Johnson (1994), maltreated children showed poorer school outcomes in general than nonmaltreated children, although cognitive outcomes were the most significantly affected. In another study by Leiter and Johnson (1997), they found a significant relationship between maltreatment and falling grades, increased absenteeism, worsening school deportment, retention in grade, and involvement in special education programs.

Eight of the children who are described in the subsequent chapters were receiving special education services when Advocacy Services began representing them. The remaining two became eligible once the representation began. The process by which children become eligible for special education services and the types of services available are described here, so that many of the interventions made on their behalf, delineated in the subsequent chapters, will have more meaning.

SPECIAL EDUCATION

At the time the U.S. Congress passed the Education for all Handicapped Children Act in 1974 (currently called the Individuals with Disabilities Act) (IDEA, 2004), over a million children with disabilities were being excluded from public school, and the million who attended public schools were receiving an inappropriate education. The purpose of the Act was to remedy this educational disenfranchisement by requiring that all students with disabilities receive a free public education, in the least restrictive environment, that is appropriate to their needs. In order to bring about the extensive changes that this law required, Congress built into the law a set of procedures for schools to follow to ensure that children with disabilities would receive an appropriate education.

Since the enactment and implementation of federal special education law, there has been great success in ensuring that children with disabilities have access to a free, appropriate, public education and in improving the educational outcomes for some children within this population (Hunt & Marshall, 2005). However, there also have been serious problems with the law's implementation, including a lack of compliance with many of its provisions by school districts around the country (National Council on Disability, 2000; Weatherly & Lipsky, 1977; Weinberg, 1997). In addition, research by Wagner (1995) shows that children with certain disabilities, such as those with serious emotional disturbance, are at greater risk for school failure, dropping out of school before graduation, and poor prospects in terms of employment and living independently once out of school. In addition, there is documentation that foster youth with disabilities experience additional problems in trying to have their needs appropriately met within both the general and special education systems (Zetlin, Weinberg, & Shea, 2006a).

What follows is a description of the procedures required by special education law along with some of the specific problems encountered by the children described in this book. A more detailed account of the problems described in this chapter, as well as how these problems were addressed, appear in the subsequent chapters devoted to each child's story.

Referral and Assessment Process

According to the current federal special education law (IDEA, 2004), all students with disabilities within a state, including children with disabilities who are homeless or wards of the state, who are in need of special education and related services must be identified, located, and evaluated. This identification process requires a variety of ongoing procedures by a school district, such as periodic screening of school children for possible disabilities, teacher referrals to determine if a student is eligible for special education, parental notification about the availability of special education services, and about the right of parents and others to refer children for an evaluation to determine if they have eligible disabilities.

Once a student is suspected of having a disability, a full and individual initial evaluation by school district personnel in all areas of the child's suspected disability must take place, typically after obtaining consent in writing from the child's parent, guardian, or appointed surrogate parent. The IDEA (2004), however, states that the local education agency (LEA) is not required to obtain informed parental consent for an initial evaluation, if the parents' whereabouts are unknown, the rights of the parents have been terminated, or the rights of the parents to make educational decisions have been given to an individual appointed by a judge to represent the child.

Areas in which a child may need assessment include social/emotional/behavioral functioning; cognitive/intellectual ability; vision and hearing acuity; health/medical status; academic achievement in reading, writing, and arithmetic; and fine and gross motor skills. The purpose of this assessment is to determine if the student has a disability as defined in the IDEA and, if so, what the educational needs are of the student (see Exhibit 2.3).

For children in foster care who have a history of being kept out of school (frequently by abusive or neglectful parents), school districts are sometimes reluctant to assess them for special education services since it may be difficult to distinguish between a reading disability, for example, and difficulty reading due to failure to attend school. This was the situation for Carlos, one of the children described in this book. At age ten, Carlos was reading at a kindergarten to first grade level.

The assessment issues for Carlos' sister, Silvia, age sixteen, were somewhat different. Although she was identified as eligible for special education on the basis of a specific learning disability in the area of reading, she was not given an adequate evaluation. Consequently, the specific nature of her reading problem and appropriate interventions to help her learn to read, after she failed to progress in this area, were not assessed. Nor was Silvia assessed to determine if she required mental health services to help her benefit from her special education program, although the school district psychologist had received records showing there were concerns in this area.

EXHIBIT 2.3.
Child Find

All children with disabilities residing in the State, including children with disabilities that are homeless children or are Wards of the State, and children with disabilities attending private schools, regardless of the severity of their disabilities, and who are in need of special education and related services are identified, located, and evaluated. . . . (IDEA, 2004, §1412(a)(3)(A))

In addition to the procedures for referring a child for an assessment, there are legal time lines within which the assessment must occur. The total time to complete an initial assessment and hold an individualized education program (IEP) meeting to discuss the results must not exceed sixty days (IDEA, 2004). What this means is that once there is written consent for assessment, the child's school district must complete a comprehensive assessment of the child and hold a meeting to discuss the assessment results within sixty days, including determining whether the child is eligible for special education services. However, if the child moves to another school district once the previous school district has begun the evaluation, the sixty-day time line does not apply for the new school district if this district is making adequate progress to ensure prompt completion of the evaluation and the parent and school district agree to a specific time when the evaluation will be completed. The new district must take into account the date on which the child was first referred for evaluation in any local education agency. Furthermore, the school district must coordinate the evaluation with the prior school or school district.

Four children in the study experienced evaluation time line violations and some of them more than once. In Silvia's case, there was a six-month delay from the time a referral was requested to the time the school district acted on that referral.

When a child who has an IEP moves to a new school district that district must provide the child with a free, appropriate education, including comparable services to those the child received in the previous school district. The new district then must conduct its own evaluation, if determined to be necessary, and develop a new IEP or continue the prior IEP. In the state where the children described in this book lived, when a student moves into a new school district, that district must evaluate the child and hold its own IEP meeting within thirty days (Special Education Programs, 2005).

Many children in foster care experience frequent residential moves (Courtney, Terao, & Bost, 2004; Eckenrode, Rowe, Laird, & Braitwaite, 1995), which was the case for many of the children described in this book. These moves usually require a change of school or school district, disrupting special education assessment time lines along with the receipt of instructional and other services.

Individualized Education Program

At the IEP meeting, based on assessment information and input from members of the IEP team, a determination is made as to whether the child is eligible for special education services (IDEA, 2004). If the IEP team finds a child eligible to receive special education services, the team then decides what goals must be addressed to meet the child's needs and what instructional program and services are required to address the goals. A child may not be placed in a special education program without having been appropriately evaluated and found eligible for special education services.

There are eleven categories of disability in the IDEA (2004) by which a child may become eligible for special education services.[1] The decision to qualify a child for special education services is a team decision, which includes the child's parent, guardian, or appointed surrogate parent and is based on relevant information provided by multiple sources (e.g., school psychologist, teacher, parent) (see Exhibit 2.4).

Two of the children in the study were eligible for special education services on the basis of having a specific learning disability and five

EXHIBIT 2.4.
Categories of Disability Under the Individuals
with Disabilities Education Act

- Autism
- Hearing impairments, including deafness
- Mental retardation
- Multiple disabilities
- Orthopedic impairments
- Other health impairments
- Serious emotional disturbance, referred to as emotional disturbance
- Speech or language impairments
- Specific learning disabilities
- Traumatic brain injury
- Visual impairments, including blindness. (IDEA, 2004, §1402 (1)(B))

were considered emotionally disturbed. One child was considered both learning disabled and emotionally disturbed, while another was identified as having both an emotional disturbance and a traumatic brain injury. Two children were considered to have multiple disabilities, with mental retardation as one of their disabling conditions.

IEP Team

The IDEA (2004) is quite clear in specifying who must attend an IEP meeting. Required participants include: a representative of the local educational agency (e.g., school district); a special education teacher or service provider (e.g., speech and language specialist); a regular education teacher if the child is, or may be, participating in the regular education environment; the child's parent; among others. At an IEP meeting for Anthony, the only people present were his special education teacher and an Advocacy Services representative. Because there was no school district representative who had the authority to commit agency resources and ensure that services would be provided, a needed service recommended by the teacher was not forthcoming (see Exhibit 2.5).

Parental Role

The IDEA (2004) is quite clear about who may sign the consent for a special education assessment and authorize the special education

---

EXHIBIT 2.5.
Required IEP Team Members

- Parents of a child with a disability
- At least one regular education teacher of the child, if the child is, or may be, participating in the regular education environment
- At least one special education teacher or service provider
- Representative of the local education agency
- Individual who can interpret the instructional implications of evaluation results
- Other individuals who have knowledge or expertise regarding the child, including related services personnel as appropriate

services for a child. These include a child's natural, adoptive, or foster parent (unless a foster parent is prohibited by State law from serving as a parent), a guardian, or an appointed surrogate parent. The law requires the local education agency or the juvenile court to appoint a surrogate parent for a child when: (1) no parent for the child can be identified; (2) the school district, after reasonable efforts, cannot discover the whereabouts of a parent; or (3) the child is a ward of the state (see Exhibit 2.6).

The surrogate parent who was appointed to represent Sharon while she was in the county emergency shelter neglected to sign the consent to have her evaluated by the local department of mental health (DMH). Consequently, when she was placed in a residential treatment program in another school district, the mental health evaluation could not be started until a new surrogate parent was appointed. By the time it was discovered that the consent had not been signed, the new residential program was no longer willing to keep Sharon in the program because of her aggressive and threatening behavior. It took placement in yet another residential program, in another school district, before a new surrogate parent was appointed for her. By this time, the time lines for her to receive a mental health evaluation were well exceeded.

EXHIBIT 2.6.
Definition of Parent

Under the Individuals with Disabilities Education Act, the term *parent* refers to

- Natural parent
- Adoptive parent
- Foster parent, unless a foster parent is prohibited by State law from serving as a parent
- Guardian, but not the State if the child is a ward of the State
- Individual acting in the place of a natural or adoptive parent, including a grandparent, stepparent, or other relative, with whom the child lives
- Individual who is legally responsible for the child's welfare
- Individual assigned to be a surrogate parent. (IDEA, 2004, §1402(23))

Instructional Placement

Special education students, according to the IDEA (2004), are to receive services that are appropriate to meet their unique needs and provide them some benefit. Both Patty and Anthony were in special education programs that did not address their disability-related needs. Patty's disability was caused by a severe head injury which left her with multiple deficits, necessitating that she have systematic training to learn (or relearn) certain skills and abilities that were within her capability; and for those she could not master, learning compensatory strategies would be required. She was placed, however, in a special education program for students with serious emotional disturbance, where no systematic skill training was undertaken.

Anthony had autistic-like perseverative behavior, communication deficits, and significant hyperactivity. His special education placement was a class for students with learning disabilities. This class required significant independence, since it was set up so that students rotated from one activity center to another. Because Anthony required a program with a high degree of structure and an emphasis on language and communication skills, which the class for students with learning disabilities did not have, he frequently was sent home from school because of his disruptive or aggressive behavior. Anthony eventually was placed in a class for students with severe language disorders, but neither the classroom teacher nor the aide had any training in addressing Anthony's behavioral needs.

John and Carlos were in general education classes without any services to address their special education needs. John, James, and Carlos were placed in special education programs with inappropriate peers, who were either lower functioning, significantly older, or extremely disruptive.

Related Services

For students who qualify for special education services, some require what are called related services (e.g., speech and language services, psychological counseling, and physical therapy). IEP teams, in addition to determining the student's eligibility for special education, specific goals to address the student's needs, and appropriate instructional placements, also must identify needed related services that assist students in benefiting from their special education programs (see Exhibit 2.7).

Sharon, although identified as having a severe language disorder, was in a program that did not have any speech and language services available. Neither James' nor Roberts' IEPs provided sufficient psychological counseling to meet their needs.

Transition Services

In recent years, the U.S. Congress became increasingly concerned about the poor school outcomes of a great many students with disabilities, such as not finishing high school, living independently, having a job, or pursuing further education after high school (Wagner, 1995). A Report of the House Committee on Education and Labor stated:

> Even for those students who stay in school until age 18, many will need more than two years of transitional services. Students with disabilities are now dropping out of school before age 16, feeling that the education system has little to offer them. (House Report, 1990, p. 10)

EXHIBIT 2.7.
Related Services

Related services, as specified in the IDEA, include the following services:

- transportation
- speech-language pathology
- audiological services
- interpreting services
- psychological services
- physical therapy
- occupational therapy
- recreation, including therapeutic recreation
- social work services
- school nurse services
- counseling services, including rehabilitation counseling
- orientation and mobility services
- medical services, for diagnostic and evaluation purposes only. (IDEA, 2004, §1402(26))

Because of this concern, specific language was added to the IDEA requiring transition services to be included in the IEPs of students who are sixteen years and older.

The purpose of the transition services is to promote the student's successful movement from school to post school activities. Transition services are to focus on a student's needs related to postsecondary education, vocational training, employment, independent living, or community participation (IDEA, 2004).

Children in the foster care system, who have no parents to guide them, are particularly in need of adequate transition services. The special education transition services should be coordinated with independent living and other services offered by CPS to help youth transition to an independent life after they exit the child welfare system.

Although transition services are essential for many foster youth receiving special education services, nevertheless, a transition plan was not added to either Robert's or Sharon's IEPs when they became sixteen. Furthermore, when transition services specifically were requested neither of them were provided any needed vocational education services.

Service Implementation

When a child's IEP specifies an instructional placement or other services, special education law (Assistance to States for the Education of Children with Disabilities, 2005) requires that the child receive this placement or services immediately. In both David's and Carlos' cases, requests for mental health referrals were agreed to by their respective school districts and the requests were written on the children's IEPs; however, in both of the cases the referrals were not made. In addition, Carlos was placed in a general education class, although his IEP specified his need for a full day, special education class. John did not receive any educational services because the new school district he entered, as a consequence of a change in his foster care placement, did not have the type of special education program he needed and that was specified on his IEP. Sharon did not receive speech and language services or one-to-one services from a specialist, although both of these services were specified on her IEP.

MENTAL HEALTH SERVICES

There is a provision in the state law (Interagency Responsibilities for Related Services [Interagency Responsibilities], 2004) where the children lived that allows school districts to refer special education students to DMH for assessment to determine if the students have mental health needs that impair their ability to benefit educationally (and that the school districts cannot appropriately serve these students through their counseling and psychological services programs). If the mental health assessors find the students eligible for these mental health services, students then may be provided, depending on their identified needs, individual, group, or family psychotherapy, day treatment, medication monitoring, or a residential treatment program.

A referral to DMH typically is requested at a student's IEP meeting. Unless the school district disagrees with this recommendation, the school district then must immediately forward the referral with supporting paperwork to the appropriate office within DMH. When DMH receives the referral, a mental health evaluator has sixty days (once the child's parent, guardian, or surrogate parent consents to the assessment) to complete the evaluation and return to an IEP meeting with the child's school district. At the IEP meeting, if the child is found eligible for mental health services, the department of mental health representative writes the mental health recommendations for services on the child's IEP, along with goals and objectives, the child's current mental health functioning, and other required information. The mental health services, once they are written on the child's IEP, are to be provided immediately, unless there are circumstances, such as working out transportation arrangements, which require a short delay.

Referrals were requested for mental health evaluations for all the children except Debra, whose developmental disability was sufficiently severe to preclude her from benefiting from psychotherapy. In David and Carlos' cases, the school personnel did not know how to make the mental health referrals. Furthermore, a major problem for many of the children was the difficulty in obtaining mental health services because of their frequent changes in residence, which sometimes placed them in new school districts. The department of mental health would then require a new referral from the new school district, adding significant time to the referral and evaluation process.

Other problems were also related to DMH's role in providing services to children under the jurisdiction of the dependency court. In John and Sharon's cases, DMH claimed no responsibility for these children and refused to provide the evaluation or services requested.

Due Process Mediations and Hearings

The IDEA (2004) requires each state to implement procedures whereby a parent, guardian, surrogate parent, or student having reached the age of majority, can challenge decisions that a school district, or other relevant agency (such as department of mental health), makes relating to the identification, evaluation, or educational placement of the child, or the provision for that child of a free, appropriate, public education. In two of the children's cases, mediations and hearings were filed for with the state Special Education Hearing Office to challenge denials of specific special education instructional placements or other services denied by school districts, a county office of education, or DMH. Mediations were held and state-level mediators helped resolve the disputed issues.

CONCLUSION

The overview of the special education process and description of problems experienced by the children should serve to set the stage for the more detailed descriptions that appear in the following chapters. Special education can provide a powerful set of services for students with eligible disabilities; however, all too often children in the foster care system do not get the services they need.

SUMMARY

The purpose of this chapter was to inform the reader that children in the foster care system receive special education services at a much higher rate than other children in the school population and provide reasons why this is the case. The chapter also delineates the major components of the federal special education law, the Individuals with Disabilities Education Act, and highlights some of the problems that the children whose cases are described in this book faced in trying to get their educational needs met under this law. This chapter provides a foundation for understanding some of the cracks that foster children face in the educational system.

Chapter 3

Sharon:
Preventing Placement
in a State Psychiatric Hospital

INTRODUCTION

As discussed in Chapter 1, if the allegations of abuse or neglect of a child are supported during the adjudication hearing, then a disposition hearing will take place to determine who should have legal custody of the child, where the child will live, and what services the child and family will receive based on what is thought to be in the best interest of the child (Badeau & Gesiriech, 2003; Weisz, 1995). A case plan is required and must include specific information such as the permanent long-term placement goal for the child and a description of the child's placement and other services (Schweitzer & Larsen, 2005). While the law is clear about what is required when the state takes custody of a child, bringing about a placement that is truly in the child's best interests is frequently difficult, as is apparent in the case of Sharon, an African-American female, whose needs did not conform to the typical placement options available. Furthermore, child protective services (CPS) has not until recently had a mandate to focus on a child's overall well being, which includes his or her education (AFSA, 1997). Attaining appropriate services for Sharon proved to be a difficult hurdle for her advocates who struggled to have her educational needs addressed in the various facilities in which she was placed.

The type of out-of-home placement preferred for any foster child removed from a parent's custody is with relatives when they are

The Systematic Mistreatment of Children in the Foster Care System
© 2007 by The Haworth Press, Taylor & Francis Group. All rights reserved.
doi:10.1300/5136_03

available, willing, and have a home that is considered to be a safe environment. The next preferred placement option is in a family home with licensed foster parents. Some foster parents take in one child who, in the ideal situation, becomes a member of the family. Some of these foster parents are looking for children to adopt and are interested only in young, healthy, and frequently, nonminority children. Other foster parents take in children, usually several, as a way of supplementing their income.

Children, like Sharon, who are older and have emotional or behavioral problems, are not likely to find a placement in a foster home and therefore, these youngsters typically will be placed in group homes. Some are small six-bed homes and others are large residential facilities with onsite special education schools and mental health services. In these group homes, rotating childcare staff are hired to care for the children. For those having more severe emotional and behavioral problems, they may find themselves placed in locked residential treatment facilities or psychiatric hospitals.

Sharon is not unlike many children in the foster care system whose significant emotional and behavioral problems make them difficult to place in stable living environments, let alone environments that will help them become productive adults. CPS frequently has difficulty finding placements that not only will accept these children, but also will keep them in the placement and treat their mental health and educational needs appropriately. Some of the children cycle in and out of group homes, psychiatric hospitals, and temporary shelters in, what often is referred to as, foster care *drift* or the *revolving door* of foster care placements (Janko, 1994). Too often, when they become adolescents, these youngsters find themselves pushed into the delinquency system and are treated as "bad kids" rather than those suffering from the consequences of not only abuse and neglect, but also, while in the custody of CPS—unstable living environments, inadequate mental health treatment, and inappropriate educational services. This chapter shows the tremendous effort involved in trying to find an appropriate living situation, school, and mental health treatment to meet the significant needs of children like Sharon. It also describes the interventions required, both to prevent an inappropriate state hospital placement for Sharon and also to prevent her entering the delinquency system.

CASE STUDY OF SHARON

Physical Abuse

Sharon began her history with CPS at age two. Her eighteen-year old mother, whom Sharon's father had abandoned during her pregnancy with Sharon, inflicted what was described in her CPS records as nonaccidentally inflicted trauma. At the time the physical abuse occurred, Sharon's mother was living with another man.

Prevention

CPS determined that Sharon was not safe living with her mother and her mother's new boyfriend and removed her from her mother's care to prevent further abuse. She was placed in the home of relatives. At first, the juvenile court did not allow Sharon's mother to see Sharon alone. Her visits had to be monitored by the relatives with whom Sharon was now living (see Exhibit 3.1).

Intervention

In an effort to reunite Sharon with her mother, but to prevent further abuse, Sharon's mother was ordered by the juvenile court to participate in parenting classes to learn other ways to discipline her. After Sharon's mother successfully completed the parenting classes, the court started allowing her to spend time with Sharon alone. Her mother's boyfriend was no longer in the picture.

Sexual Abuse

When Sharon was almost five, CPS recommended that Sharon be allowed a ninety-day home visit with her mother and the juvenile court judge agreed. If things went well during this visit, there was an excellent possibility that Sharon would again live with her mother on a permanent basis. What occurred, however, during this ninety-day visit was that a male member of the family sexually abused Sharon. Her uncle was suspected, but this was never confirmed. CPS reports described the abuse as severe and ongoing.

EXHIBIT 3.1.
Placement History

Age	Placement	Maltreatment	School
2 yrs.	Relative	Physical Abuse	N/A
4 yrs. 9 mos.	Parent		N/A
5 yrs.	Legal Guardian	Sexual Abuse	Elem. School
9 yrs. 1 mo.	Psychiatric Hospital		Hospital School
9 yrs. 4 mos.	Legal Guardian		Elem./Jr. High
13 yrs. 2 mos.	Psychiatric Hospital		Hospital School
13 yrs. 4 mos.	Emergency Shelter		Shelter School
13 yrs. 6 mos.	Group Home		N/A
13 yrs. 6 mos.	Emergency Shelter		Shelter School
13 yrs. 7 mos.	Moontree Residential		NPS
14 yrs. 4 mos.	Emergency Shelter		Shelter School
14 yrs. 5 mos.	Hutchinson House		NPS
14 yrs. 9 mos.	Lighthouse Residential		NPS

N/A = No records available.

Elem. = Elementary School.

Jr. High = Junior High or Middle School.

NPS = Nonpublic School (i.e., a private special education school).

Intervention

To try to ensure that Sharon's home visit with her mother would be successful, the court required that Sharon receive psychological counseling. The counseling took place at a hospital pediatric project whose focus was child abuse. Sharon's therapy consisted of one counseling session each week for forty-five minutes. It was the staff at this pediatric project that discovered, during counseling sessions, that Sharon was being sexually abused.

Prevention

Child protective services removed Sharon permanently from her mother's care and placed her in foster care.

Placement with a Legal Guardian

Sharon lived until early adolescence in a home with five other girls and a foster mother who became her legal guardian. Her school records show she repeated her kindergarten year because the school staff felt she was not ready academically, socially, or emotionally for the first grade. When she did matriculate to the first grade, the records describe her as having difficulty getting along with peers, having a poor self-concept, and requiring a significant amount of individual attention by her teacher. Sharon was described as being easily distracted, frequently struck out aggressively against other children, and displayed little evidence of self-control. She was evaluated by the school district and subsequently determined to be eligible for special education services. Shortly after, she was placed in a special education class for children who were considered to have a serious emotional disturbance. Without the history of abuse and lack of appropriate treatment and care, it is likely that Sharon would not have had the severe emotional disturbance that made her eligible for special education services (see Exhibit 3.2).

Sharon remained in special education classes for the next several years, with her defiant, aggressive, tantrum-prone behavior only increasing with time. At the age of nine, Sharon's guardian, unable to contain her behavior, had her admitted to a child psychiatric unit at the county hospital where she remained for three months. The conclusion reached by the psychiatric social worker at the hospital was that Sharon was not only suffering from probable unresolved emotional conflict stemming from the multiple incidents and types of abuse, but also from the lack of opportunity to resolve this conflict through a reparative relationship with her guardian. According to the psychiatric social worker, the guardian failed to effectively place

EXHIBIT 3.2.
Emotional Disturbance

1. The term means a condition exhibiting one or more of the following characteristics over a long period of time and to a marked degree that adversely affects a child's educational performance:
   - An inability to learn that cannot be explained by intellectual, sensory, or health factors.
   - An inability to build or maintain satisfactory interpersonal relationships with peers and teachers.
   - Inappropriate types of behavior or feelings under normal circumstances.
   - A general pervasive mood of unhappiness or depression.
   - A tendency to develop physical symptoms or fears associated with personal or school problems.
2. The term includes schizophrenia. The term does not apply to children who are socially maladjusted, unless it is determined that they have an emotional disturbance. (Assistance to States, 2005, §300.8).

limits on Sharon's acting-out response to stress, periodically rewarding her with solicitous care for her instances of dramatic misbehavior, and encouraging her misbehavior outside the home by minimizing it and defending her against those who reported it.

Over the next several years, Sharon's behavior in school did not seem to change much, even though she was now taking medication to address her behavioral problems. She remained in special education classes for students identified as having serious emotional disturbances. She still had problems with her peers, although, by the sixth grade, she was described as having found less aggressive outlets for her anger. Even so, when she was upset, she still cried, became extremely loud, and tipped over chairs. Academically, she was reading at a third grade level.

Shortly after starting junior high, Sharon was once again hospitalized by her guardian for hyperactive and aggressive behavior at home. Apparently, her acting out behavior began to intensify. While Sharon was hospitalized this time, her guardian decided she no longer wanted to provide a home for her. Consequently, the legal guardianship was terminated and CPS reinstated its jurisdiction in the case.

Intervention

To reduce the effect of the trauma of sexual abuse, Sharon received psychological counseling throughout the first year she was placed in the home of the caregiver who became her legal guardian. In addition to the individual therapy that Sharon received, she and her guardian attended a couple of family therapy sessions together. Sharon's guardian also received a half dozen parent conferences to assist her in managing Sharon's behavior at home and school. It was not until almost three years later, however, when her guardian felt Sharon's behavior at home had become unmanageable, that psychological counseling again was initiated.

During Sharon's first hospitalization, the psychiatric social worker tried to address the guardian's ineffectual parenting skills in family therapy sessions that included both the guardian and Sharon. While there seems to have been progress, with the guardian gaining some insight into why she had trouble setting clear limits for Sharon or showing anger towards her, once Sharon was discharged from the hospital the counseling sessions were discontinued.

What Had Gone Wrong?

One of the ongoing concerns in child welfare is finding adequately trained caregivers for children with extremely difficult behaviors. Sharon's guardian apparently needed ongoing training and support to help her set appropriate limits for Sharon.

Determining an Appropriate Placement Option

After the legal guardianship was terminated, Sharon then spent two months at the county emergency shelter followed by eleven days at a small group home before she was returned again to the emergency shelter because of her behavior, which was described as assaultive and destructive. This time Sharon remained at the emergency shelter for a month and a half before moving to the locked residential treatment facility where I first met her, almost nine months later.

When Sharon was fourteen, the juvenile court appointed Nancy Shea, senior attorney at Advocacy Services, to represent her. The purpose of this representation was to determine whether the state hospital for those with severe mental illness was appropriate and, if not, to help identify a placement environment that would be stable for her.

Intervention

The first time I met Sharon, she was living in a locked residential facility for youth with severe emotional disturbance. Sharon's placement by CPS in this locked residential facility included individual, group, and family psychological counseling in an attempt to reduce her acting out, aggressive behavior. Psychotropic medication was prescribed as well and she lived in a twenty-four-hour structured environment.

I was visiting the facility to talk with staff members about their recommendations for Sharon's treatment and to spend some time talking with her about placement options. Before talking with Sharon, however, I had met separately with an administrator and with Sharon's therapist. The clinical administrator, a man in his mid-forties, described Sharon as a young woman who, after a nine-month stay at the facility and a regimen of behavioral and cognitive therapy, along with trials of various psychotropic medications, was no closer to controlling her impulsive, aggressive behavior than when she started the program. She was, in his view, desperately searching for an identity, feeling lost when she was part of a group and only able to find herself by being loud and challenging. While ruling out a diagnosis of schizophrenia or "prepsychosis," the administrator was recommending that she be placed in the state psychiatric hospital, on a unit with adolescents who were considered too mentally ill for a less restrictive placement in the community. CPS was set to follow the placement recommendation of this administrator.

Sharon's therapist, a young man, was somewhat more hopeful about her prognosis. He described a young woman who had been progressing adequately in her treatment and then started regressing. He speculated that the regression was related to the onset of puberty or her failed attempts to establish a sustaining relationship with her mother in family therapy sessions. He described several family therapy sessions in which Sharon's mother became furious, yelling and screaming while denying any responsibility for Sharon having been abused.

Then I met with Sharon privately for about twenty minutes. I found her to be a pretty young woman with an athletic build, polite and engaging. Sharon communicated in no uncertain terms that she did not want to go to the state hospital. Nancy, her attorney, had already discussed with her that under state law she could not be placed in the state hospital unless she agreed to it or was considered a danger to herself or others or gravely disabled (Lanterman-Petris-Short Act [LPS], 1968). No one was suggesting that she met the criteria for involuntary placement in the state hospital.

In light of Sharon's teetering on the brink of a state hospital placement, her attorney requested a court-ordered psychological evaluation. The psychologist who was appointed to evaluate Sharon concluded that placing her at the state hospital would lead to irreparable psychological damage, since the state hospital was for individuals who are chronically psychotic and for whom no available treatment is effective. It was his belief that Sharon was treatable, that she had shown him that a therapeutic alliance was possible. He stated in his report to the court that her anxiety, fear, and rage were a consequence of having been abused and abandoned by everyone of significance to her. He thought it was natural, under the circumstances, that she had developed a pervasive suspiciousness and mistrust of others, as well as extreme hypersensitivity to control.

The placement recommendation of this psychologist was for a residential program where the residents live in cottages with house-parents or permanent staff. This recommendation, however, was made with the assumption that Sharon's only likely chance for success was that if she had a therapist who was able to continue treating her several times per week for years, even if she changed where she was living. The psychologist saw Sharon's treatment as a re-parenting process in which the therapist would be greatly tested by her for a long period of time.

Advocacy Considerations

Sharon's court-ordered attorney took her responsibility seriously to have services provided to Sharon that were in Sharon's best interest. To carry out this obligation, she engaged in the following activities:

- She did not automatically accept a recommendation to have Sharon placed in the most restrictive living environment, a state hospital for those too mentally ill for community placement.

- She requested and received a court order from the juvenile court for a psychological evaluation to determine whether a restrictive hospital placement was in Sharon's best interest (see Exhibit 3.3).
- She conferred with her client, Sharon, about the placement options and explained her legal rights to her about needing her consent for state hospital placement (see Exhibit 3.4).
- By engaging in these activities, Sharon's attorney was able to influence the CPS case plan and placement recommendation for Sharon.

The Stopgap "Solution"

The psychologist's report and Nancy's advocacy kept Sharon out of the state hospital; but they unfortunately were not able to produce the recommended placement and treatment option. Upon discharge from the locked residential facility, Sharon entered the emergency shelter since there were no other identified placements that had agreed to accept her. She had cycled through the emergency shelter several times before. This time she remained at the emergency shelter for eight months, time enough to establish a fairly close relationship with her classroom teacher and the school psychologist, before being moved again to another residential facility.

Intervention

Sharon was accepted into a new CPS program, called Stopgap, which provided an additional $2,000 per month per child above the typical group home rate for hard-to-place children. Within a month, at age fourteen and five months, Sharon left the emergency shelter to enter a residential program that was to provide her with intensive mental health treatment. Part of the Stopgap philosophy was that the

---

EXHIBIT 3.3.
Court Orders

Request a court order for a psychological evaluation to help determine an appropriate placement for a foster youth with serious emotional and behavioral problems.

EXHIBIT 3.4.
Conferring with a Client

Remember that the foster child is your client. Let the child know his or her legal rights and possible placement options. Seek input from the child regarding placement preference.

residential facilities, which participated in the program, would use the extra funding they received for a specific child to provide specialized and individualized services to that child. This was the condition under which the generous funds would be allotted. In addition, the facilities would have to agree not to discharge the children for their extremely difficult and sometimes dangerous behavior, since the extra funding was to be used to provide one-to-one aides, additional therapy, or whatever was seen to help reduce or contain problematic behavior. The point and hope of the Stopgap program was to insert a permanent wedge into the revolving door thereby bringing to a stop to the children being continually kicked out of foster homes, group homes, and residential facilities, and returned on a regular basis to the emergency shelter, sometimes for extended stays. The problem for the county was that the emergency shelter was not set up to be a permanent placement for a child and it was extremely expensive (i.e., $6,000 per month of county dollars) to keep a child at the emergency shelter for more than thirty days.

Sharon's program at the Stopgap residential facility, called Hutchinson House, included individual psychotherapy three to five times a week, group therapy five times a week, and participation in therapeutic recreational activities. She attended school in a self-contained special education class near her living quarters.

Sharon's initial relationship with the staff at Hutchinson House got off to a fairly good start. But, very quickly, she became demanding, insisting on one-to-one attention from the staff and becoming extremely jealous when this attention was not available. Gradually her behavior became defiant and verbally aggressive, accelerating to extensive property damage. She threw a desk over in the classroom, threw nail polish on the walls, ripped a telephone cord out of the wall, broke a ceiling light fixture, tore a door off its hinges, threw a chair through the window, and sprayed a fire extinguisher over the living quarters. Eventually, she fled the facility without permission and was picked up by the police who had been notified by Hutchinson House's program staff of her absence. The police took her to another residential facility that was providing respite care for the Stopgap program. Sharon spent the next three weeks going back and forth between Hutchinson House and the respite program. Her behavior at the Hutchinson House program seemed to be at an all-time low.

Finally, being unwilling to endure Sharon's continued aggressive behavior, the staff at Hutchinson House made it clear that she was no longer welcome in the program. A meeting was held where Nancy asked CPS to provide additional services to the residential program in order to keep Sharon there. However, the director of the facility was insistent upon pressing charges against Sharon for throwing the chair through the window. Both Nancy and the CPS worker in charge of the Stopgap program tried to convince the director to drop the charges against Sharon. The director finally did agree to drop the charges on the condition that Sharon would be removed permanently from the program, which is what happened.

What Had Gone Wrong?

Had this program required more of Sharon than she was capable of handling? She had not been verbally abusive or aggressively destructive during her eight months at the emergency shelter. The emergency shelter provided a fairly low-stress environment for the children who stayed there. Sharon also felt cared about by her teacher and the school psychologist at the shelter. Sharon's lack of trust in this new placement is evident by her statements that her therapist was racist.

Upon Sharon's admission to Hutchinson House, all aspects of the intensive mental health program started at once. The written concerns of the psychologist who had evaluated Sharon to determine whether she was appropriate for the state hospital helped to explain her behavior at this facility. The psychologist indicated in his report that Sharon would not be able to handle insight-oriented psychotherapy for some time. What was necessary for her, he believed, was for trust to be developed over several years before Sharon would be able to enter into a therapeutic relationship in which "an interpretation of her defenses or her psychodynamic history" could occur. He felt that she was terrified of intimacy, untrusting and guarded, which made sense since the most important individuals in her life had either been abusive or abandoned her. He also reported that she was extremely anxious and frightened and that her anger was a defense against her fear. It also was noted in the report that Sharon did not have the "ego strength" to be able to hear criticisms from her peers without feeling extremely injured or responding with extreme hostility.

Stopgap and Delinquency

Intervention

The revolving door of placement continued as Sharon entered into another residential Stopgap program, which was called Lighthouse Residential Center. She had some familiarity with this program, since it was one of the programs that provided respite for her from the last program.

The therapeutic component of the residential program consisted of individual therapy for the residents and a weekly group meeting on the living unit. Individual therapy also was available on a crisis basis. A mental health professional or intern provided the individual therapy, and the group meeting was conducted by the childcare staff.

On the day after admission to Lighthouse, Sharon had a serious run-in with a teacher, which almost landed her in the juvenile delinquency system. Sharon's version of the story was that while waiting outside her assigned classroom (not far from her living unit), she was touched on her shoulder by her teacher, a man whom she had not met before. She said he had no right to touch her and push her toward the classroom, so upon entering the classroom she started swearing at him. At some point, he tried to grab her and she started throwing chairs and books at him to try to keep him away. Sharon claimed the teacher grabbed her arms and forced her to the ground in an attempt to physically restrain her. But, she said, he was unable to effectively restrain her, leaving her legs free to kick him in the knees.

The "official" version of this incident, which appears in an incident report of the residential facility and was written by the classroom aide, indicates that after being directed into the classroom, Sharon threw three chairs, one of which hit one of the other students. When she was asked to leave the classroom, Sharon then went to the teacher's desk and started throwing books and papers that hit the teacher in the face. As Sharon was about to throw containers filled with paper at the teacher, he held her arms so that he would not get hit. The report goes on to say, Sharon slipped on all the books and papers on the floor and, when she was down, she kicked the teacher repeatedly on his legs. She was trying to swing at him as well but he held her arms.

After this incident, the teacher filed delinquency charges with the police against Sharon for assault and, subsequently, took a disability leave from teaching. Sharon, in a somewhat self-righteous tone, tried to disparage the teacher's attempt to restrain her, telling me that it was against the policies of the facility for someone on the staff to try to restrain a resident by himself, without the support of at least one other staff member.

I requested a meeting with the residential and school program staff at Lighthouse to discuss what appeared to be a policy of the facility to encourage the staff to press charges with the police against the youngsters in their care. While I in no way condoned Sharon's assaultive and destructive behavior, I was concerned that this facility was collecting a significant amount of money to not only house, but to provide an appropriate therapeutic program for youngsters who had serious mental health problems.

At the meeting, various staff members argued that they needed to be able to threaten potentially assaultive youngsters with being sent to juvenile hall in order to maintain them safely in their program. In Sharon's case, the staff claimed that the involvement of the probation department would give them more leverage with her. There seemed to be no understanding that the facility had been given additional funding to individualize a program for Sharon.

The other issue we discussed at the meeting was why a male teacher would touch a female adolescent student whom he did not know. Even though it was not recorded in the incident report, it seemed to be general knowledge that the teacher had touched Sharon prior to her outburst. There was no satisfactory response given by the staff as to why this had occurred.

What Had Gone Wrong?

Any teacher who taught at this facility's school should have had an understanding of the type of problems the children placed there had

had before, and had been sensitive to how to approach a new student. One might have hoped that those who were to work with Sharon would have reviewed her past records and put together a plan on how to address her needs before she arrived. Had this occurred, perhaps this assaultive incident with the teacher might have been avoided.

Furthermore, even though CPS had initiated a special program for youngsters like Sharon—the Stopgap program—the residential facilities that participated did not have an understanding of what it entailed. Unfortunately, CPS did not seem to have enough control over the facilities (or, at least, was not organized to take the control) to make them comply with the philosophy of the Stopgap program.

Delinquency or Dependency

Since delinquency charges were filed against Sharon—a youngster who was under the jurisdiction of CPS—this triggered the requirement of a written report jointly prepared by CPS and the probation department. The question that had to be addressed in the report was whether to retain Sharon's status with CPS or transfer her case to the probation department. If the transfer occurred, then Sharon would be considered a delinquent rather than a dependent. Her case still would be under the jurisdiction of the juvenile court, but it would be in delinquency court rather than dependency court.

The immediate problem, however, was how to get the required report written. The difficulty here was that Sharon did not have a CPS social worker. When her residence changed from one part of the county to another, she was supposed to be assigned a new social worker. But, this had not occurred.

The date for the delinquency court hearing was set for May. Surprisingly, Nancy, Sharon's dependency court attorney, was not notified of the date. I just happened to hear about it while visiting Sharon at Lighthouse. Because Nancy had to be in dependency court that day on another case, I was the one from our office who went to Sharon's delinquency court hearing. I showed up at 8:00 a.m. on the day of the hearing, since there was no way to know what time a particular case would be heard. Everyone whose case was to be heard in delinquency court that day had to check in by 8:00 a.m. and then just sit and wait. The waiting room was large and bare except for chairs with hard backs and seats lined up in rows. On one side of the room, behind a glass barrier was an attendant with whom everyone had to check in; on the other side was a small snack bar. Other than that, the only decoration was a large clock on the wall.

Sharon arrived shortly after I did, accompanied by a woman from Lighthouse. I learned that this staff person was not someone whom Sharon had met before that morning. I was informed that everyone else from the facility was busy. Sharon was pretty nervous at first, not being quite sure what the outcome would be of the delinquency court hearing. She had never met the delinquency court attorney who would be representing her in the hearing. This was par for the course. The court-appointed attorneys for delinquency court had enormous case-loads, and typically reviewed the case records and meet their "client" on the day of the hearing, sometimes just an hour before.

I tried to keep Sharon calm. After several hours of nervous chatter, she settled down and became sleepy. The room was warm. She put her head down on my lap like a young child and appeared to sleep for a while. We continued waiting while names and courtroom numbers were announced over a loudspeaker and small groups of people, usually an adolescent and an adult, left the waiting room. The hours passed slowly.

At about 12:30 p.m. the snack bar abruptly closed. It was at this point that I learned that Sharon had not eaten breakfast that morning and the staff person with her had neither food for her lunch nor money to buy her something to eat. We also realized that the snack bar was now closed for the day and that we would have to drive to get anything to eat.

The delinquency court was in a fairly remote, desolate area, which was not unusual since it was attached to a juvenile detention facility. I drove us all toward the town and luckily found a small convenience store where I purchased food for Sharon and then quickly drove back in time for the afternoon court session to begin. I was somewhat concerned about how Sharon's behavior would be as the afternoon wore on because she had missed her noon dosage of medication. The staff person was not given any of Sharon's medication to bring with her in case the court hearing did not take place until the afternoon, as was the case.

At about 2:00 p.m., Sharon's delinquency court attorney came to talk to us. He told Sharon that the judge who was to hear her case was tough, but fair. He cautioned her to watch her language and answer the judge's questions in a very respectful manner, saying "yes, your honor" and "no, your honor." I introduced myself to the attorney, having briefly spoken to him on the telephone several days earlier. He seemed fairly certain that the judge would change Sharon's status to delinquent as of this hearing and that there was not much he or anyone could do about it. He did not seem to be up on the state statute that required a jointly written report by CPS and probation before a change to the delinquency system could occur for a dependent like Sharon.

The appointed delinquency court attorney left us alone and went away to represent another client before Sharon's case was called. By this time, Sharon was visibly upset. Her voice was becoming louder by the moment. She said nobody could tell her what to say to the judge; she'd say "whatever I f***ing feel like." She insisted that she would not say "yes, your honor" or "no, your honor." The judge would "just have to f***ing accept me as I am;" she was not going to change for anyone. I started worrying; concerned that Sharon's behavior would quickly escalate to verbal and physical aggression. I was not sure what to do, but I just quickly started talking to her. I told her that of course, she had to be herself in front of the judge, but the Sharon I knew was a caring, sensitive, lovely young woman. I told her I knew she liked to be treated with respect and that she preferred to treat others with respect. After I went on like this for some time, I could tell that Sharon was starting to calm down. She was listening carefully to me. She finally said she would treat the judge respectfully if the judge treated her respectfully, but that she would not say "yes, your honor" or "no, your honor." I let her know that it would be fine if she simply answered "yes" or "no" to questions that required those answers.

We heard Sharon's name and the number of the courtroom announced over the loudspeaker and quickly went down the hallway to the courtroom. By the time we were ushered into the courtroom, Sharon's delinquency court attorney was seated at one of the tables in front of the room facing the judge, with the prosecuting attorneys from the county at another table facing the judge. There was a row of seats several yards behind them where the bailiff motioned us to sit.

When Sharon's name was called by the judge, she answered politely that yes, she was present. I breathed a little easier.

The judge asked Sharon's attorney if there was anyone in attendance from the residential placement facility or CPS who could provide some background in this case. The staff person with Sharon indicated that she was from the residential facility, but that she only drove Sharon to the courthouse and did not know anything about her history. The judge then turned to me and I told her my name, the law office I worked for, and the attorney from my office who represented Sharon in dependency court. The judge indicated that she knew Nancy, Sharon's dependency Court attorney, having recently moved from dependency to delinquency court. I could tell that we were off to a good start. I told the judge the facts in the case, as I knew them. The judge ultimately continued the case, setting the next court hearing three months later, to allow sufficient time for CPS and probation to write the required joint report before any placement decision was made about Sharon. Sharon had a few more opportunities to answer the judge's questions and did so politely. It was now late in the afternoon and we were all relieved to have this over for the time being.

What Had Gone Wrong?

Sharon arrived at the delinquency court ill equipped to handle the day's activities. No one from CPS or the residential treatment facility made sure someone was with Sharon who could provide the relevant information needed by the delinquency court judge. Furthermore, Sharon was not provided any psychological support by sending her to the hearing with someone she did not know and her physical needs were not provided for either in terms of food or medication.

Advocacy Considerations

It turned out to have been extremely important that I attended Sharon's delinquency court hearing, both to support Sharon and to provide crucial information to the judge. It seems obvious that an adult who is knowledgeable about a foster youth's history and, hopefully, trusted by the youth, should attend delinquency court hearings, if that should be necessary.

A Search for a Social Worker

Sharon had been placed at Lighthouse Residential Center since the beginning of February, and it was now the end of May and her case was just being transferred from one CPS regional office in the county to another. When the case was finally transferred, a social worker still was not assigned. At the end of June, after many attempts to have a social worker appointed, Sharon's attorney decided to call the director of the regional CPS office who assured her that a social worker would be assigned immediately. The assignment finally was made not too long after. The problem then was getting the new social worker to review the case file and write the report required by the delinquency court. It took several weeks and many calls before the social worker was sufficiently knowledgeable and, still more time, until she found time to write the report.

Consultation with Probation

At the time we were trying to encourage Sharon's new CPS worker to complete the report in time for the August hearing, we also had been talking with the probation officer assigned to the case to apprise him of Sharon's history and current situation. We scheduled a meeting with the probation officer to talk further with him about the case. At the meeting, he told us since the teacher and residential facility insisted on pressing charges in this case, and also because Sharon had a fight with another resident where charges were pressed, the minimum he could recommend was informal probation for Sharon. What this required was that Sharon would be on informal probation for six months and would be able to maintain her dependency status at this time, so her Stopgap funding would not be jeopardized. If, in this six-month period, Sharon did not violate any of the rules of the Lighthouse program, then, when she returned to court, the informal probation would end and her dependency status would simply continue. However, if Sharon violated the rules of the residential facility in this period of time, she would end up on regular probation and enter the delinquency system. We understood informal probation was the best we could hope for Sharon when she returned to delinquency court. We were uncertain whether she would be able to follow the rules of the residential facility without any violations for six months.

Advocacy Considerations

If Sharon ultimately became a delinquent, the negative consequences for her would be considerable: (1) Nancy, her current court-
appointed attorney with whom she had developed a relationship
would no longer represent her, since Nancy had been appointed by
the dependency court; (2) Sharon would lose her Stopgap status and
funding; (3) the most serious problem, however, would be that she
would be viewed and treated as a delinquent rather than a youngster
whose behavior was seen in the context of a history of abuse and abandonment. Any infraction of rules could land her deeper and deeper
into the delinquency system, with the possibility of her ending up in
the Youth Authority—the most secure prison in this system.

Inadequately Trained Childcare Workers

Sharon's dependency court attorney and I brainstormed how to
stop Lighthouse Residential Center staff from pushing their residents
into the delinquency system for behavior that was indicative of a history of serious emotional disturbance. We learned that Sharon was
not the only youngster with whom they had tried this approach. The
local police department told us that the staff at Lighthouse, in addition to pressing charges against the residents themselves, continually
brought in the residents to press charges against each other.

We also were concerned about the lack of training of some of the
staff members. One incident was quite telling. Sharon called our office one afternoon and I took the call, being the only one in the office
at the time who worked on her case. She was obviously quite upset
and seemed like she needed someone with whom to talk. She started
to tell me what had occurred, but before she got very far, I heard what
appeared to be a struggle and then one of the staff from Lighthouse
was on the phone. He told me he had taken the phone away from
Sharon and would not let her continue the conversation with me because she was not being truthful about how terrible her behavior had
been or what had occurred at the residential facility. I told him that
Sharon had called her attorney and had a right to a private conversation. At that point, the staff person hung up the telephone.

Another incident also troubled us. We learned about a fight that
Sharon got into with another resident. One of the staff tried to stop the

fight by shouting and ordering them to stop. When Sharon would not listen, this staff person started swearing at her, using profanity, and spit in her eye. We were somewhat consoled that this staff person was fired the next day, but continued to be troubled about what appeared to be a general lack of training of the childcare staff who were with the residents on rotating shifts.

What Had Gone Wrong?

CPS placed children in particular residential treatment facilities because their social workers believed the programs were designed for those with extremely serious emotional and behavioral problems. But, in fact, for some of these residential treatment facilities there was not much of a program at all and that was why the staff resorted to this continuous process of pressing charges against the residents. It appeared that no one within CPS had evaluated the quality of the total program provided, including the mental health treatment. The social workers, under tremendous pressure to find placements for children on their caseloads, were simply relieved to have the beds that were available, particularly for difficult youngsters like Sharon.

Advocacy Considerations

Nancy wrote a very strong letter to the County Commission on Children and Families, an appointed body that monitors the work of CPS, describing the problems at this residential facility. The Commission immediately began an investigation (see Exhibit 3.5).

Attending to Sharon's Educational Needs

As an agency appointed to represent children who have been abused or neglected, one of Advocacy Services' main concerns, in addition

EXHIBIT 3.5.
Reporting Concerns with Residential Programs

Write detailed letters to relevant agencies and commissions to initiate investigations regarding suspect practices at residential treatment facilities.

to an appropriate living situation, was the quality and appropriateness of education the children received. Consequently, once Sharon was admitted to Lighthouse Residential Center, I contacted the on grounds nonpublic school at the facility that she would attend.

The First IEP Meeting

I requested an individualized education program (IEP) meeting to review Sharon's educational program since, because of her change of residence, she now was in not only a new school but also a new school district. This IEP meeting took place a month after Sharon first entered the residential facility.

At the meeting, the principal of the school noted and wrote on Sharon's IEP that she had a severe language deficit, based on an evaluation that was done while Sharon was at the emergency shelter. This evaluation concluded that she had a language disorder "characterized by significant difficulty in paying attention to spoken language and properly interpreting relationships between words in sentences." The recommendation for Sharon was to receive speech and language services, in addition to her classroom special education program. Surprisingly, however, the principal did not authorize any speech and language services for Sharon. Thinking of this as somewhat strange, I requested that Sharon receive speech and language services. What I learned then was that this school and residential facility did not have a speech and language specialist on staff. The school district representative at the meeting recommended a reevaluation of Sharon's speech and language needs, which gave the nonpublic school some time to determine if there were any specialists from the school district available to provide the service for Sharon.

No one, at this time, knew the whereabouts of Sharon's mother; consequently, a surrogate parent had been appointed for Sharon by the school. A surrogate parent is able to authorize special education services for a child who does not have a parent or whose parents' whereabouts are unknown. In addition, a surrogate parent is supposed to advocate on behalf of the child for an appropriate school program. The surrogate parent appointed for Sharon had never met her nor had reviewed her school records. However, the surrogate parent did attend the IEP meeting.

Before the meeting ended, I requested a referral for a mental health evaluation for Sharon in order to determine whether the mental health services she received from this residential facility were adequate, given our concern that the facility did not appear to have much of a therapeutic program. The surrogate parent signed the required form allowing the referral to proceed as well as the reevaluation of Sharon's speech and language needs.

Within a month after this IEP meeting, Sharon was evaluated by the school district's specialist who also recommended that Sharon receive speech and language services. Two months after Sharon had entered this residential facility, she again had speech and language services on her IEP. However, speech and language services were not provided for her for another three months.

What Had Gone Wrong?

Speech and language services, which legally should have started immediately upon Sharon's entrance into the school program at this facility, took five months to begin.

Advocacy Considerations

The surrogate parent's lack of familiarity with Sharon did not prove to be a problem in this case because I was present at the meeting and knowledgeable about her needs. However, without a knowledgeable surrogate parent for a child at an IEP meeting, the needs of a student with a disability may not be properly addressed (see Exhibit 3.6).

EXHIBIT 3.6.
Surrogate Parent Responsibilities

One state requires a surrogate parent to meet with the child who the surrogate is appointed to represent at least once. The surrogate also may meet with the child on additional occasions, attend the child's IEP meetings, review the child's educational records, consult with those involved in the child's education, and sign any consents relating to the child's IEP. (Calif. Gov't Code §7579.5(d))

The Second IEP Meeting

At the second IEP meeting, the DMH evaluator reported that he had completed a mental health evaluation of Sharon, but that his agency would not provide any services for her since she was receiving mental health services from the residential facility already. My hope had been that DMH would make a determination as to whether the mental health services that Sharon was receiving at Lighthouse Residential were adequate to meet her educational needs and, if not, supplement those services or recommend needed changes. This was my understanding of what the law required (Interagency Responsibilities, 2004). I also wanted DMH to provide some case management services, particularly in the event that the current residential facility no longer wanted Sharon in its program.

There was another issue that I decided to broach at this meeting. My concern was that Sharon had not progressed academically for several years. Her reading, math, and written language scores were quite low; although, it was clear she had the ability to achieve at higher levels in these subject areas. No doubt, her emotional and behavioral problems were detrimental to her learning in addition to the frequent changes of where she lived; but I was not sure that was the whole picture. In various reports and observations of her in school, there was mention of the fact that she needed someone working with her one-on-one for her to do her work. Consequently, I requested that a specialist work with Sharon—someone with specific training in teaching youngsters with learning problems. I wanted someone who would work with her individually to try and identify the specific problems she had in advancing in reading, math, and written language and the ways that these problems might be addressed.

The other set of circumstances I believed that warranted having a specialist work with Sharon was there had not been a regular teacher in the classroom since she injured him on her second day of school at the facility. Furthermore, she was frequently out of the classroom on school days, either wandering the halls or sent back to the living unit because of inappropriate behavior at school. The other concern I shared was that when anyone from my office observed Sharon's classroom, the students were walking around and leaving the classroom at will and those who remained were usually talking loudly, and not about any classroom-related subject.

The principal did not know how to handle the request I made for an educational specialist for Sharon. Consequently, she suggested that we schedule yet another IEP meeting where she would invite the director of the residential program and representatives from the local school district.

Advocacy Considerations

The importance of having DMH's involvement in future place- ment decisions for Sharon was that the mental health agency had de- veloped a considerable expertise in matching a youngster's mental health and special education needs with available facilities. However, it became clear that it was futile to pursue DMH's involvement in Sharon's case any further at this IEP meeting. The evaluator who at- tended did not have the authority to alter purported policy for the agency (see Exhibit 3.7).

The Third IEP Meeting

The next IEP meeting took place about a month later. The classroom situation at the facility's on-grounds school had not changed. To my surprise, the IEP team actually recommended on Sharon's IEP that she would have the use of an educational specialist to work with her indi- vidually for three months to determine if it made a difference in her ability to learn. Specific goals were written for the sessions with the specialist. The one crucial issue that was not decided at this meeting was who was going to provide or pay for these services. The program

---

EXHIBIT 3.7.
Individualized Education Program (IEP) Meetings

Do not continue to argue a point at an IEP meeting if the person who has the authority to make decisions is not present. Adjourn the meet- ing and reschedule at another time. It is always a good idea prior to an IEP meeting to let the school district or other relevant agencies know the issues you want to address and the people who you would like to be present.

director of the facility made it clear that neither the Lighthouse residential program nor the on-grounds nonpublic school planned to pay for these educational services. The school district also refused to pay; the district representative argued that its contract with this nonpublic school required the school to cover all needed related services of its students. This meeting ended without resolving this issue.

Advocacy Considerations

It had become clear that nothing would be resolved by having another IEP meeting. Consequently, I initiated the special education appeal procedures on Sharon's behalf, which are guaranteed in federal and state special education law (IDEA, 2004; see Exhibit 3.8 here).

The Mediation

Several weeks after I had filed for a state special education hearing, a mediation conference took place (which is the way the process was set up in the state). The setting for this mediation was in a conference room at the Lighthouse Residential Center. The key players were present—representatives from the school district, the residential facility, the on-grounds school, the department of mental health, and I from our office.

After the mediator described how the mediation process works and the guidelines she wanted us to follow, it was up to me to present the issues in the case, which I did. After my presentation, each party in the case was given an opportunity to add additional information. The mediator then divided us up (putting us in different rooms) so she could talk with each party in the case separately.

After several hours of "shuttle diplomacy," with the mediator going back and forth between the various parties trying to hammer

---

EXHIBIT 3.8.
Resolving Disagreements at IEP Meetings

Initiate a due process hearing if having another IEP meeting is unlikely to resolve a disagreed upon service for a child with a disability.

out a document to which all could agree, eventually she informed us there was an agreement. The mediation agreement stated that the department of mental health would provide case management services and act as a liaison with CPS to ensure that the mental health services that Sharon received were appropriate. In addition, the school district would complete a comprehensive psychoeducational assessment of Sharon so that assessment information about her would be up-to-date and complete, and hopefully provide insight into Sharon's learning problems. The nonpublic school agreed to provide one-to-one educational services for Sharon three times per week. The school principal would be the specialist providing these sessions, since she had a special education credential to teach students with learning disabilities and also the experience working with those with serious emotional and behavioral problems.

Advocacy Considerations

While I had some reservations about whether the school principal would be able to provide the intensive educational services satisfactorily, I generally was pleased that the mediation process produced the results it did. However, I also was saddened that the time and effort of so many people were required to bring about results that should have been easily forthcoming several months earlier.

CONCLUSION

Why did Advocacy Services expend time and energy trying to correct problems in a residential facility and their on-grounds school, rather than request that Sharon be transferred to another facility? The reason, unfortunately, was there was no other place in the county to send her that would be any better. Most of the residential facilities simply would not admit her because of her behavior, which we were told was—on a regular basis—aggressive, destructive, and sometimes assaultive. Sharon most likely would have benefited significantly from being the only child in a foster home of a couple who had received sufficient training to cope with her. These foster parents would need adequate monetary compensation so there would be no need to take in other foster children. They also would need crisis intervention and respite services readily available along with ongoing counseling and support. Sharon would need the type of psychotherapy that was recommended in the psychological report that kept her out of the state hospital. Services like these—often called wrap-around services or therapeutic foster care—are available in certain parts of the country. But in the county where Sharon lived, they did not exist at that time.

Given the severity of the emotional and behavioral problems that many abused and neglected children experience today, appropriate placement options for these children must be developed and be available. Large-scale residential facilities with inadequate mental health services, poorly trained staff, and schools that are at best baby-sitting services will not do. Services must be child-focused and of high quality. Otherwise, we are expending large sums of money to simply maintain these youngsters until they become eighteen and are on their own. What we find then is they are unemployable, and end up on the streets or in our jails and hospitals (Cook, 1994; Courtney, Dworsky, Terao, Ruth, & Keller, 2005; McMillen & Tucker, 1999). There are other options. We must choose them for the children and for the society.

SUMMARY

The purpose of this chapter was to describe how a foster child's court-appointed attorney was able to prevent her placement in a state psychiatric hospital, but then struggled to find the type of placement and services that had been recommended for her. The chapter shows how special programs set up to provide stability for difficult-to-place youngsters may fail to achieve their results because the goals of the program are not well understood by those who are funded to implement them and there is no mandatory accountability. In addition, special education appeal procedures may be required to improve the special education services a youngster receives at an on-grounds non-public school at a residential treatment facility.

Chapter 4

John:
Struggling to Stabilize Placement
with a Parent

INTRODUCTION

The U.S. federal law requires that child protective services (CPS) develop a case plan for children removed from the custody of their parents for abuse or neglect (Adoption Assistance and Child Welfare Act [AACWA], 1980). For the first twelve months that a child is under the jurisdiction of the juvenile court, reunification with the child's parents often is the goal of the case plan. When such reunification plans are appropriate, CPS typically requires that the parents make certain constructive changes in their lives in order for their children to be returned to them. These changes might include taking a parenting class, completing a drug rehabilitation program, or getting a job and a permanent place to live. Whether the child can be returned safely to the parent is a decision that will be made by the court with input from CPS. If the child is still in out-of-home placement by the twelve-month review hearing, the case plan must then identify permanent placement for the child. Reunification with the parents still can occur after the twelve-month court hearing, but CPS may no longer be working actively to reunite the child with the parent at this point.

John's case was well past the required twelve-month hearing when Advocacy Services became involved. But John had never given up hope of reuniting with his mother. CPS still was working with John's mother to help bring about their reunification, but not as actively as it might have been. There were still many requirements that his mother had to meet to have John back with her.

The Systematic Mistreatment of Children in the Foster Care System
© 2007 by The Haworth Press, Taylor & Francis Group. All rights reserved.
doi:10.1300/5136_04

CASE STUDY OF JOHN

Suspected Child Abuse

John's parents never married and his father denied paternity. Although John was born full term and his developmental milestones were normal, his mother found his behavior difficult since infancy—very hyperactive and easily excitable.

When John was eight, he was taken into police custody after a suspected child abuse report. John's mother admitted to having beaten him severely on numerous occasions, becoming extremely frustrated and overwhelmed at not being able to control his aggressive behavior. As a result, it seems that John had developed a pattern of running away from home as a means of escaping the physical abuse. Also, by the time he was eight, he had been unsuccessful in several school programs, including a class for students with serious emotional disturbance that included a counseling component. Apparently, the services provided had little effect at controlling his behavior. Consequent to this placement, he attended a nonpublic special education school paid for by the school district.

Intervention

CPS placed John in a psychiatric hospital for two months to try to contain his running away and other seemingly uncontrollable aggressive behaviors. After his discharge from the hospital, however, his behavior had not improved. He still was assaulting others and continued running away, only now, he also threatened suicide (see Exhibit 4.1).

CPS Assumes Custody

Prevention

Several months after John returned home from the hospital, CPS assumed custody and he became a dependent of the juvenile dependency court. CPS had removed him from his mother's custody because of her inability to handle him and her ongoing use of severe physical punishment to try to control him, which CPS considered abusive. On this last occasion, when John's mother had beaten him and tied his hands with an extension cord, CPS removed him from her care.

EXHIBIT 4.1.
Placement History

Child's Age	Placement	Maltreatment	School
8 yrs.	Hospital		Hospital School
8 yrs. 2 mos.	Parent		NPS
8 yrs. 5 mos.	Foster Home	Physical abuse	Elem. School
8 yrs. 7 mos.	Emergency Shelter		Shelter School
8 yrs. 8 mos.	Schaffer Residential		NPS
9 yrs. 10 mos.	Emergency Shelter		ES School
10 yrs. 2 mos.	Ellison Group Home		Elem. School
10 yrs. 3 mos.	Emergency Shelter		Shelter School
10 yrs. 5 mos.	Georgine Group Home		NPS
10 yrs. 8 mos	Emergency Shelter		Shelter School
11 yrs. 2 mos.	Stockton Group Home		Kellon/NPS
12 yrs. 1 mo.	Emergency Shelter		Shelter School
12 yrs. 6 mos.	Group Home		
12 yrs. 6 mos.	Emergency Shelter		Shelter School
13 yrs. 3 mos.	Foster's Group Home		
13 yrs. 6 mos.	Emergency Shelter		Shelter School
13 yrs. 7 mos.	Applegate Residential		Spec. Ed. School
14 yrs. 1 mos.	Parent		NPS

NPS = Nonpublic School (i.e., a private special education school)

Elem. = Elementary School

Spec. Ed. School = Public Special Education School

Intervention

CPS placed John in a foster home where he lasted only two months before the foster family decided they could not deal with his out-of-control behavior. CPS then placed John in the county emergency shelter until there was an opening for him in a residential treatment facility for boys who were considered emotionally disturbed.

While at the emergency shelter, John underwent a psychological evaluation. He communicated to the psychologist who performed the evaluation that he had run away from the foster home because other boys who were living there had beaten him up. He indicated that he liked being at the emergency shelter because he felt safe; in addition, he acknowledged that he refrained from running away from the shelter because he wanted the privileges and points he received for acceptable behavior.

On the psychological evaluation, John's measured intelligence was in the average range and, according to the psychologist, there was no substantial evidence suggesting an organic basis for his problems. However, he showed poor impulse control, had an inability to sit still, had considerable anxiety, and was extremely fearful. He was diagnosed with *adjustment disorder with mixed disturbances of emotions and conduct* and possible visual perceptual motor problems. The recommendation of the psychologist was placement in a mental health residential facility that provided good, positive-oriented behavior management and individual counseling. The psychologist's opinion was that John needed protection from others and from his own impulses until he gained better control over his fears.

Placement in a Residential Treatment Facility

Intervention

John was placed almost immediately at Schaffer Treatment Center, a residential facility like the one the psychologist had recommended. Shortly after his arrival, he quickly reverted to his pattern of violent outbursts and running away whenever he felt upset or angry. He started receiving individual psychological therapy and also the medication he had been placed on when he was hospitalized to help control his behavior was changed. The individual therapy focused on John role-playing appropriate responses to actual incidents that occurred on the living unit. He also entered into a behavior contract with his therapist agreeing to reduce his aggressive behaviors toward others. During his stay at the residential treatment facility, John made slow and steady improvements in his behavior, which his therapist and other staff felt were connected to elevations in his self-esteem. He was able to eliminate his running away behavior for six months. While the aggressive behaviors continued, they declined in frequency.

Shortly after placement in this residential treatment facility, John was evaluated by the local school district in the area. John was in the third grade and four months shy of his ninth birthday at the time. The school psychologist found that John had a minor perceptual motor delay, was quite needy of adult interaction, and was unable to cope when angry or upset and, instead, acted out. The report also noted that he was aggressive toward others in class about three times per week, made derogatory comments or inappropriate gestures to students and teachers, and demonstrated dramatic mood changes. His academic functioning was about one to two grades below his grade level. At his individualized education program (IEP) meeting following this evaluation, John's special education classification of emotional disturbance was continued and the school district agreed to fund his nonpublic school placement at the residential treatment facility.

During the year and two months that John was placed at Schaffer, his mother visited him infrequently. He complained that his mother would make promises to pick him up, and then would not show up. One of the problems for John's mother was she did not own a car and public transportation to the facility from her home was extremely difficult. It took a tremendous amount of time to get there and still did not take her right up to the facility. Consequently, John's mother did not participate in any family therapy sessions during his stay at this residential treatment facility.

Finally, without a specific known cause, John's behavior rapidly deteriorated. He began to run away again, and his aggressive episodes increased dramatically in frequency and severity. During one episode, he threw a brick, hitting his therapist's back and causing serious injury. He also threw rocks at the facility staff and at peers, all at close range. The clinical staff decided he was a danger to others and needed a more highly structured setting than they could provide where he could be monitored more closely.

What Had Gone Wrong?

When CPS placed John at Schaffer's Treatment Center, his mother's ability to visit him and participate in his treatment should have been of prime consideration. The case plan, at this stage, still was for John to reunite with his mother when his aggressiveness and running away behavior decreased and when his mother demonstrated competent parenting skills.

The likelihood of this treatment plan being actualized was significantly diminished by John's mother having so much difficulty securing transportation to the residential treatment facility. In addition to her not having a car, she had little money, and public transportation was almost nonexistent. CPS should have provided her with taxicab vouchers in order for her to continue to be a part of her son's life by participating in the treatment this residential facility offered (see Exhibit 4.2).

Abuse in the Child Care System

After John was discharged from Schaffer Treatment Center, he went to the county emergency shelter for four months and then spent one month in the Ellison Group Home, where his aggressive behavior could not be contained. He was returned to the emergency shelter for two months, and then was placed in the Georgine Group Home where a staff member took extreme measures in trying to deal with his difficult behavior. After unsuccessful attempts to contain John's aggression, an employee of this group home drove John more than fifteen miles away from the home and dropped him off in the woods,

---

EXHIBIT 4.2.
Preparation for Reunification

If family reunification is likely, actively involve the child and parent in ongoing psychological counseling. Ensure that the parent has adequate transportation to get to the counseling sessions.

for all intents and purposes abandoning him. The police found John wandering the streets at night and returned him to the emergency shelter at 1:30 a.m.

What Had Gone Wrong?

It is an understatement to say that the Georgine Group Home had not provided adequate training to its staff on permissible and effective ways to discipline children with difficult-to-control behavior. Unfortunately, a high percentage of childcare staff at group homes are paid low wages so people without much education or training take these jobs.

Advocacy Consideration

CPS notified the state agency that licenses and monitors group homes. This agency investigated the incident of John having been abandoned and ordered the home to be closed. Rather than contesting the decision, the group home voluntarily ceased operating (see Exhibit 4.3).

Advocacy Services Appointed

About this time, Advocacy Services was appointed by the juvenile court to represent John for the purpose of stabilizing his placement. The plan for the time being, with which John agreed, was to keep him at the emergency shelter since his violent behavior made it difficult to find a group home or residential treatment facility that was willing to accept him. It also was deemed important that a placement be found that would not quickly discharge him when his behavior became difficult or dangerous.

When the law office first started representing John, Nancy, Advocacy Services senior attorney, requested a court order from the juvenile

---

EXHIBIT 4.3.
Licensing Violations

Report violations of licensing requirements in group homes to the appropriate licensing agency.

court for a neuropsychological evaluation for John. Within a month, the evaluation was completed indicating that John had mild hyperactivity, was somewhat distractible, had an impulsive response style, and his mood was mildly anxious. He had deficiencies in short-term memory and was diagnosed with developmental reading, arithmetic, expressive and receptive language, and spelling disorders. The recommendations from the psychologist included an educational program that focused on strengthening his basic academic skills, a referral to a speech and language pathologist for an evaluation of his language capabilities, and placement in a small structured learning environment with direct supervision to help reduce the negative effects of his emotional disturbance on learning (see Exhibit 4.4).

Advocacy Services' senior attorney also decided to try to find a law firm interested in bringing a personal injury suit against the group home whose employee had abandoned John in the woods, since Advocacy Services did not do this type of law. Letters were sent to several law firms and one expressed interest in investigating the possibility of such a lawsuit.

Advocacy Considerations

Nancy requested a court order for a neuropsychological evaluation of John in an attempt to better understand his behavioral and learning problems. She hoped to understand as fully as possible the causes of his behavior so as to plan appropriately for him.

A Period of Residential Stability

Placement at the emergency shelter was successful in stabilizing John's living situation for the time being. In fact, he received honors for his behavior in the living unit.

**EXHIBIT 4.4.
Court Orders**

Request a court order for a psychological or neuropsychological evaluation to help with program planning for a difficult-to-place youth.

After six months at the emergency shelter, however, John once again was placed in a group home, called Stockton, and this time he started attending Kellon Middle School, the local middle school in the community. But, not surprisingly, placement at the middle school turned out to be more than John could handle and, as a result, he ended up hitting and biting a teacher. Subsequently, the school district recommended that John again be placed in a nonpublic special education school, believing his behavior was too difficult to be managed safely on a public school campus. He was in the sixth grade and eleven years and two months at this time. John remained in the nonpublic school and Stockton Group Home for almost a year before his behavior again became out of control and dangerous.

Intervention

In addition to John's placement in another nonpublic school for students with emotional and behavioral problems, most importantly, while at the Stockton Group Home, he and his mother started receiving counseling together with the goal of working toward their reunification. He also was going on overnight visits with her on a regular basis. At that time, however, John's mother did not have a place of her own and was living in a small apartment with her own mother. The plan for John to live with his mother required that she get a job and a place of her own, which she was planning on doing.

Several events conspired to destroy John's tenuous well-being. First, his mother did not secure employment or rent an apartment according to schedule, which meant that John's returning to live with her permanently could not occur as quickly as he had anticipated. Second, the weekly overnight visits he was having with his mother stopped around the same time.

What Had Gone Wrong?

In order to facilitate John's reunification with his mother, his CPS case had been transferred from one social worker and office (i.e., permanency planning) to another social worker and office (i.e., reunification). However, this change took over two months to be completed and during this time, John did not have a social worker overseeing his case. It appears that this disruption in a social worker overseeing the case led to the cancellation of the home visits.

Residential Stability Ends

An event occurred at school that seems to have been the last straw in the collapse of John's fragile stability in this treatment facility. While at school, a "friend" asked John to hold his art supplies for him, which John did. The "friend" then proceeded to falsely accuse John of having stolen the art supplies and, John subsequently was accused of stealing by the art teacher. Consequently, and not surprisingly, John ended up feeling set up by his "friend." This incident, along with his disappointment related to his mother, seemed to send John into a tailspin. He did not have the coping skills to deal with the situation rationally and, instead, kept the anger bottled up inside. He became enraged and refused to go to the school. When he did go, he acted out aggressively.

John ran away from school early one morning. The police found him wandering later that night and returned him to the group home at about 4:00 a.m. That same morning the childcare staff at the group home decided that the proper course of action was to send John to school, even though he was completely exhausted from his night away. They felt that requiring him go to school even though exhausted would act as negative reinforcement for running away, what they saw as constituting a "natural consequence" of that behavior. However, once at school, John ran away again, but returned to the group home on his own volition about 8:00 p.m. the same night.

The following morning John again was taken to his nonpublic school, but was required to talk with his therapist before being readmitted to the class. John communicated to the therapist that he did not want to be in school. The therapist contacted the group home, but no one was able to come and pick him up. After many hours and an encounter with the school's behavior specialist who discussed with him the behavioral requirements for readmission to class, John, feeling unable to comply with these requirements, simply walked out of school. One of the teachers at the school followed him. John then picked up a large rock and threw it in the teacher's direction, shattering a window. John's therapist came outside to try to deescalate John's behavior.

The therapist eventually was able to calm John and the staff from the group home had arrived by then and transported him back to the home.

Prior to this incident, arrangements had been made with John's mother to meet with John and his therapist at the group home that afternoon. So, when John returned to the home, his mother already was there. John did not want his mother to know about the incidents that had taken place at school. Nonetheless, the therapist explained to John's mother what had occurred and mentioned John's feeling of rejection by his mother as precipitating John's behavior. When John heard this, he stormed out of the office in a fit of rage, picking up a plastic milk carton and throwing it at the therapy room's window. Once outside, John started throwing rocks at windows, staff, and the vans belonging to the group home. He swung a broomstick at the staff member who tried to get close to him, and pulled the telephone wires out of the wall. Although John was large—five feet seven inches and two hundred pounds at the time—several of the staff eventually were able to get behind him and restrain him. He was brought inside and given crisis intervention to calm him.

The group home staff wanted a CPS social worker to come to the group home and transport John back to the emergency shelter. However, no one at the CPS knew who John's current social worker was, and his previous social worker was unwilling to assume this responsibility. By the time that CPS was able to determine who John's current social worker was, it was well after hours and John was sound asleep.

Within a week, John's behavior again was out of control and dangerous, thus precipitating a call to the police. The police took John to the county psychiatric hospital for an evaluation of his dangerousness. When he was not deemed to be a danger to himself or others (Lanterman-Petris-Short Act, 1968), the police transported him to the emergency shelter.

What Had Gone Wrong?

The group home staff apparently pushed John too hard in requiring him to go to school after having been out all night. Whatever was bothering John and causing him to run away was not dealt with by simply sending him to school.

Why did the hospital refuse to admit John as an involuntary patient? The state law governing such evaluations requires that the person being evaluated demonstrate dangerous behavior to himself or others at the time of the evaluation. The fact that the person may have been dangerous previously or is likely to be so again in the future are not grounds enough for hospitalizing the person involuntarily.

Return to the Emergency Shelter

At the juvenile court hearing the following month, John indicated to the judge that he wanted either to remain at the emergency shelter or to live with his mother. The determination was that he would remain at the emergency shelter for the time being since there was no other suitable placement for him. For close to a year, other than the day spent at another group home, John remained at the emergency shelter.

While the emergency shelter did not have the option of throwing John out for his aggressive behavior, my colleagues and I at Advocacy Services had concerns about the emergency shelter as an ongoing placement for him. First, he was not receiving sufficiently intensive special education services to meet his academic needs. He spent two sessions per week (twenty to thirty minutes each) receiving one-to-one instruction from a special education teacher. The rest of the time, however, he was in what the school at the emergency shelter called a modified regular education class. While the class size was small—the day I observed there were nine students (although, the numbers could grow significantly when the population of the shelter increased)—John had a hard time in this setting. He did not seem to understand the simple work that was being asked of him. He fidgeted at his desk and was verbally abusive to the other students. When the class went to the school library, on the walk there, John separated himself totally from the other students and walked alone. He looked quite distressed. The classroom teacher said to me, "John doesn't deescalate easily and therefore needs a one-on-one aide with him [in school]."

The teacher indicated that John required a one-on-one aide for behavioral reasons. However, he also seemed to require an aide at this point to function academically. When John spent time out of the classroom working one-on-one with the special education teacher on vowel sounds, he smiled and almost seemed happy, and stayed focused. However, even when the special education teacher had John working on the computer by himself, he again became extremely fidgety, and had difficulty sitting still in his chair.

While at the emergency shelter this time, John received a psychological evaluation. It increased our concerns about John's educational placement at the emergency shelter school. This evaluation was a mandatory three-year evaluation under special education law. While John's intellectual capability was still considered to be in the average range of intelligence, he had severe delays in all academic areas as well as deficits in the content and form of his language usage. His academic performance had taken a nosedive since his last evaluation. John was in the seventh grade at this time.

The second concern we, at Advocacy Services, had with the emergency shelter was that John was not receiving ongoing mental health services. He met with the school psychologist for twenty to thirty minutes weekly where he mostly played cards and other games with her. While John generally liked this arrangement, no one was working with him on the serious issues that greatly affected his ongoing well being and ability to live successfully in the community. The recent psychological evaluation underscored John's need for more intensive mental health services. In completing the tests that comprised much of the evaluation, the school psychologist found John to have what she called an "impulsive response style." In addition, John made angry sounds to himself when he felt he had made an error and then became tearful. She reported that he judged himself harshly. The psychologist relayed that John was having significant difficulties following the program in the living unit. He bothered his peers to such an extent that they would hit him. He then would not fight back but, instead, would break into tears. The psychologist reported that while John appeared well based in reality, he gave what she called "free association type responses" and did not appear to understand many of the questions she asked him. Consequently, his responses seemed inappropriate. He also displayed some unusual behavior for his age, such as rocking his body back and forth. The psychologist's opinion was that John was locked in a cycle of misunderstanding, anger, distress, and self-blame. During the evaluation, John told the school psychologist that he did not consider any of the many placements in group homes or residential treatment facilities he had been in to be any good and that what he really wanted was just to be with his mother.

The IEP meeting that followed John's psychological evaluation resulted in the same school services he previously was receiving that were not meeting his needs. No in-depth psychological counseling or other mental health services were provided. Consequently, Nancy and I decided to contest the services offered to John and try to gain educational services we thought would be more appropriate. In order to do this, we filed for a hearing with the state Special Education Hearing Office. However, five days after we filed, John was removed from the emergency shelter and placed in another group home. This move from the emergency shelter was in violation of a standing court order.

Advocacy Considerations

When John was placed at the emergency shelter this last time, Advocacy Services' Senior Attorney requested and was granted a court order from the juvenile court that John should not be removed from this placement without her agreement. Nancy's thinking, in requesting this court order, was that she did not want John to have to endure another change of placement unless there was some assurance that his placement would last. However, CPS violated this court order, with no apparent repercussions for the agency.

In an attempt to secure intensive mental health services for John while at the emergency shelter, Advocacy Services contacted the department of mental health (DMH) to request the reinstatement of the type of mental health services that John had received in his previous placement. The DMH Program Head refused to reinstate the previously received mental health services, even though these services had been on his IEP, and, instead, required that a new referral be made by the education agency that ran the school at the emergency shelter. A new referral should not have been required under state law (Interagency Responsibilities for Related Services, 2004). Therefore, John was further left without the mental health services he was entitled to even though he desperately needed the services. In addition, it was fairly certain that the emergency shelter would not go along with a new referral for these mental health services. At John's IEP recent meeting at the emergency shelter, I requested such a referral. But as I had anticipated, it was turned down. The county education agency claimed that it was not a school district and this meant it had no obligation to make such referrals. Nancy and I knew that this was a violation of both federal and state special education law (IDEA, 2004; Interagency Responsibilities, 2004).

We requested a special education hearing to contest the denial by DMH of reinstating mental health services and the denial of the county education agency of making a new mental health referral. We also contested the denial of additional time for John with the resource specialist teacher. However, the removal of John from the emergency shelter and placement in yet another group home made our request for a special education hearing on these issues moot. Since the new group home was in another part of the county, John now had a new school district responsible for him. Thus, the county education agency that ran the school at the emergency shelter no longer had any responsibility for him. This was just one more crack in the system for children in foster care like John.

Another Group Home Placement

When John left the emergency shelter, he was placed in yet another group home called Foster's Group Home. He lasted there for three months before the staff decided that they no longer could handle his constant running away and aggressive behavior. John now was thirteen and a half years old.

Two weeks into his stay at this group home, John was given a psychological evaluation. An interesting, but perhaps not surprising, finding of this evaluation was that John's scores on an intelligence test had dropped from those of his previous tests. His overall intellectual functioning was no longer in the average range, but in the low average range. His score on the verbal scale was in the borderline range (between low average and mild mental retardation). The psychologist astutely acknowledged on the evaluation report that "[t]he lowered verbal IQ probably resulted from his failure to have adequately benefited from his schooling." This was an understatement, given the many changes of homes and schools that John had experienced, and not to mention his poor psychological state much of the time. He was functioning academically, according to the evaluation, at the beginning third grade level in spelling and math and at the beginning fourth grade level in word recognition. He was described as aggressive toward peers, defiant, hostile, disobeying rules, stealing, and destroying property as well as appearing to suffer from depression. The psychologist also found that he had a great deal of anger that was the result of unresolved issues related to his history of neglect and feelings of abandonment.

Early in his stay at Foster's Group Home, John broke his ankle during a skating outing. Two weeks later, when John was upset, he cut off the cast. His broken ankle did not slow down his running away very much. Since, within a month, he was leaving the facility and staying away for days at a time, requiring the police to find him out wandering the streets and bring him back. Relying on the police to contend with John's running away put John in jeopardy of being classified as a delinquent. At this point, Nancy stepped in to try to prevent John's case from being transferred to the juvenile delinquency court.

Advocacy Interventions

It did not take much advocacy on Nancy's part to stop the group home staff from calling the police whenever John ran away. What she did was to let them know that she would help bring about a change of placement for John. Nancy's ongoing contact with the group home staff was important. Without that, it was likely they would have continued calling the police whenever John left the facility without permission and he would have ended up in the delinquency system. As it happened, the group home staff stopped making police reports and ultimately seemed satisfied in the knowledge that they would not have to continue to deal with John's difficult and dangerous behavior much longer (see Exhibit 4.5).

Stopgap Program and Enrollment in School

Intervention

John was returned to the emergency shelter and within two weeks, he was accepted into the CPS Stopgap Program. It is a program for

---

EXHIBIT 4.5.
Maintaining Contact

It is important for a foster child's attorney to maintain ongoing contact with appropriate staff members at the child's placement.

hard-to-place foster youth that gave certain residential treatment facilities additional funding to house and provide therapeutic services
to these difficult youngsters and, most importantly, not terminate their
placement when problems arose. This was the same program that
Sharon was in. But as we saw in the previous chapter, the program did
not have the intended results of stabilizing her placement. The results
were not any better for John.

The first hurdle with the Stopgap placement was getting John into
school. The Stopgap residential treatment facility in which John was
placed, called Applegate Home, did not have an on-grounds school.
So theoretically, the youngsters placed there should have attended a
school program in the local school district. The problem, however,
was that the school district was small. Therefore, the Coordinator of
Special Education stated quite decisively that the district did not have
an appropriate program for students like John, who were designated
as having an emotional disturbance. Consequently, the local school
district would not enroll John in school. The director of the residential program complained to me that none of the youngsters placed in
her facility were allowed to enroll in this school district, since they all
had some behavioral problems.

The school district referred these youngsters living in this residential treatment facility to a county education program that had specific
special education programs for students with certain disabilities, in
this case, those with serious emotional disturbance. This process might
have worked out well if students were immediately enrolled in the
county school program. Needless to say, these referrals took a very
long time, and leaving the students out of school frequently for up to
three months.

Seemingly, the problem was that the school district took several
weeks to a month to put the referral together and send it off. For some
reason, on receiving the referral, the county education program assumed it had a sixty-day timeline to assess and possibly place the student in a program. If the county program administrators determined
that they did not have an appropriate program for the referred student,
the referral was sent back to the local school district to figure out
what to do with the youngster. This added many more months to the
student being out of school. We, at Advocacy Services, viewed this

referral procedure as a violation of federal special education law and one more way that children in foster care got the short end of the stick.

What Had Gone Wrong?

The local school district immediately should have enrolled John, and the other students placed in this residential facility, in a district school program. In John's case, the district clearly was required to provide him a comparable school program to the one described in his IEP from the emergency shelter (Special Education Programs, 2004). The IEP stated that John was to be placed in a regular education class with pullout services from a resource specialist twice a week. This type of program existed in the school district. If the district felt that John needed more intensive services, it could have held an immediate IEP meeting in order to provide him additional services. The district might have provided a full-time aide, increased his time with a re-source specialist, or developed a behavior plan to proactively deal with his behavioral problems. The district then would have had some assurance that there were services and a plan in place to handle John's behavioral problems if they arose. At that point, the district could have made a referral to the county education program, but John would have been in school the entire time and in a school program considered, under the law, a less restrictive placement option (IDEA, 2004).

Another problem in this case was the timeline used by the county education program when a school district made a referral to this agency. Under state law (Special Education Programs, 2005), in reality, the sixty-day timeline only applies to initial assessments to determine if a child has a qualifying disability in order to receive special education services. There was no doubt that John had a qualifying disability and he had an IEP that stated such.

Advocacy Considerations

I knew there was no way the local district was going to enroll John in one of its school programs. The Coordinator of Special Education was absolutely adamant on this point. While I might have initiated a hearing or filed a noncompliance complaint to try to contest the unilateral decision of the Coordinator, I decided instead to try to expedite the process with the county education agency. I thought the county's program was probably the better option for John at this point. Consequently, I contacted an appropriate administrator with the county education agency. I let him know that John had been in a county education program in his previous placement, when he was in the emergency shelter, and that his current IEP was from that school program. "Couldn't you," I asked "simply use John's current IEP from the emergency shelter school and immediately enroll him in your program?" The administrator agreed to do that, but first wanted to have an IEP meeting at the school in which John was to be enrolled.

I showed up at the IEP meeting thinking that it would be a quick meeting and that John automatically would be enrolled in this school. This particular county school specialized in programs for students identified with serious emotional disturbance. What I learned at the IEP meeting, however, was that the administrator of this program was concerned about John's potential for aggressive behavior. He was concerned whether his behavior was too volatile for the only classroom at the school with an opening for students his age. This classroom already had other boys in it with explosive behavior. I explained to the IEP team that John's aggressive outbursts primarily were related to his disappointment over his mother's failure to do what CPS required so that he could live with her. With that explanation, the administrators of the school decided to accept John and enroll him immediately (see Exhibit 4.6).

Another positive outcome from this IEP meeting was that a referral was made to DMH to initiate an assessment of John's mental health needs and then, hopefully, provide him needed services. This was the referral I was unable to bring about while John was at the emergency shelter.

EXHIBIT 4.6.
Choosing an Advocacy Strategy

When there is more than one advocacy strategy available to achieve your ends, determine which course of action will be most effective and time-efficient.

Stopgap Program and John's Escalating Behavioral Problems

John was unhappy in Applegate Residential Center. His desire to be with his mother was so strong that his anger often overcame him. He broke windows and damaged desks, sofas, and chairs in this residential facility. The staff had a hard time containing his aggressive behavior toward them and he also struck out at the other residents in the facility. After a particularly difficult outburst of aggression, the staff at the facility filed a police report on John for property damage.

Advocacy Considerations

Worried that the police report might land John in the delinquency system, Nancy reminded the residential facility administrator that the facility was receiving a substantial amount of money to provide John the level of support he needed to contain his difficult behaviors. Filing a police report against John did not qualify as providing him this support. The director of the residential facility ultimately agreed to drop the charges against John but on the condition that he would be removed from this facility and found another place to live. The Stopgap program failed again to stabilize a placement of a difficult-to-place foster youth.

Placement with His Mother

John finally got his wish and that was to live with his mother. However, he was placed in her home without any counseling or school services in place for him. I discussed with John's mother the importance of counseling for John and that I would help her get these services in place if she wanted. She indicated, however, that she would seek counseling for herself and John through her church. I let her know that if those counseling services did not work out, I would help her find other services. John's mother also told me that she had placed John in a nonpublic school not too far from where she lived.

About a month later, I contacted John's mother again to see how things were going. At that time, she told me that she and John no longer were in counseling because she was unable to pay for it. I let her know that I would try to get some mental health services set up for her and John as part of John's IEP so she would not have to pay for them. In order to do this, I knew that DMH would require a new referral from the current school district where John's mother lived. My first step was to contact a Senior Psychologist at the school district. In contrast to the small school district in which John's last residential placement was located, this district was extremely large and one with which I had had considerable working relations. I let the Senior Psychologist know that we needed to initiate a mental health referral for John and that it had to be done quickly in order to try to maintain John at home with his mother. This psychologist acted quickly and beyond the call of duty. He sent another school district psychologist to John's mother's home in order to obtain her signature on the form so that the referral could be initiated. After obtaining the signature, the Senior Psychologist sent the referral packet to the DMH office that was in charge of processing the referrals and evaluating the mental health needs of the respective students. The Senior Psychologist also indicated on the referral that an IEP meeting would be set up within thirty days to put the mental health services on John's IEP in accord with state law (Special Education Programs, 2005).

At the same time that the mental health referral was being processed, I decided to observe John in the nonpublic school where he was enrolled. I had some concerns about this particular school program and wanted to see whether it was meeting John's needs. During an observation at this school, I decided my concerns were justified. The academic program at this school was weak and did not provide John the kind of academic stimulation that he needed; the kind of stimulation that would keep him from falling further and further behind academically. There were few books or other materials at this school and the teachers that I observed did not have teaching credentials.

After leaving this nonpublic school, I called John's mother and shared some of my concerns about the school with her. I discussed with her that there were other nonpublic schools that might provide a better education for John and I wanted to see whether they had openings. I assured her that no change in John's school placement would take place without her and John's agreement.

I called some nonpublic schools in the area that I knew had decent academic programs and also would provide John the kind of psychological support that would help him be successful. Two of the schools had openings. My next step was to contact a nonpublic school specialist from the school district to discuss the possibility of changing John from one nonpublic school to another. This is where I ran up against a roadblock. The nonpublic school specialist would not initiate a change of school placement for John because of her concern about John's past disruptive behavior.

Unfortunately, before I decided whether and how to try to bring about a change in school placement for John, John was removed from placement at his mother's home and returned to the emergency shelter. John's behavior, within a relatively short time, had deteriorated and he was showing angry and somewhat aggressive behavior toward his mother. John now was much larger and stronger than when they last had lived together. His mother felt that she could not handle John's aggressive behavior and wanted him removed from her home.

What Had Gone Wrong?

It made no sense to me that John had been placed at home with his mother without CPS making sure all needed services were in place in order to give this arrangement its best chance of success. Good, regular mental health services should have been in place at the time John was placed with his mother. In fact, John's mother should have been receiving mental health counseling to help prepare her for the issues with which she undoubtedly would have to deal once John was with her. It also would have been a good idea, at least temporarily, to have a mental health professional come into her home to try to help maintain and stabilize John's placement with his mother. These types of counseling services certainly would have been less expensive than other placement options for John.

Advocacy Considerations

Once John was placed in his mother's home, I tried to obtain mental health services for him and his mother through the IEP process. The reason I chose that route was because there were no other easy options to obtain the intensive mental health services that John and his mother required. If John and his mother went directly to a department of mental health clinic intending to use their Medicaid benefits as payment, they would have been put on a waiting list since there were not enough mental health professionals working at these clinics in relation to the demand. Those who had diagnoses of serious mental illness, such as schizophrenia, major depression, or severe bipolar disorder, were more likely to be seen first. If John and his mother eventually made it off the waiting list and started receiving services, they most likely would have been seen in therapy twice a month at the most (see Exhibit 4.7).

Another consideration was that the mental health services that could be accessed through the IEP process should have been readily available to John and have provided him and his mother a range of service options (e.g., individual therapy, family therapy, medication monitoring) and level of intensity (e.g., twice a week) they needed.

The problem, however, was that John did not remain in a living environment long enough to have the mental health referral processed. Each time CPS moved John to a new place to live, he was in a different school district. DMH required that a new referral for mental health services be initiated each time John was moved into a new school district. Consequently, John was never able to receive the benefit of these services.

CONCLUSION

John had a desire to live with his mother. He had feelings of anger and abandonment when his mother did not follow through with the requirements of CPS so he could live with her. This jeopardized any chances of stabilizing a out-of-home placement option for him. However, when the time arose for CPS to allow John to be placed back in his mother's care, careful planning and ensuring that necessary

EXHIBIT 4.7.
Home of Parent Placement

Ensure all necessary supports are in place, such as enrollment in an appropriate school program and mental health counseling, prior to placement of a child with emotional and behavioral problems back with his parent.

services were in place did not happen. Another factor that worked against stabilizing John's placement with his mother was the difficulty of getting ongoing consistent mental health treatment for him. DMH had a process in place that worked to the detriment of youngsters in foster care, like John, who had trouble remaining in a foster care placement long enough to complete the referral and assessment process for mental health services. The fact that a different referral process could not be instituted for these hard-to-place foster youth showed more concern for the bureaucratic nature of DMH and the school districts than for troubled youth like John.

SUMMARY

The purpose of this chapter was to describe how efforts by child protective services (CPS) ultimately sabotaged John's reunification with his mother. John longed to be placed back with his mother and had considerable anger at her for not doing what CPS required to bring this about. CPS, however, then placed John in a residential treatment facility that was difficult for his mother to get to from her home. Consequently, she did not see him on a regular basis and they did not receive the family mental health therapy they needed.

After several unsuccessful out-of-home placements, John finally got his wish to be placed back with his mother. However, CPS did not prepare adequately for this placement, and he arrived at his mother's home without any mental health services or school services in place for him. Without supportive services in place for John and his mother, John's behavior problems quickly escalated and his mother requested his removal from her home.

Chapter 5

James:
Stabilizing Placement with Relatives

INTRODUCTION

The families and children that come to the attention of child protective services (CPS) present complex needs that typically require the provision of services from multiple agencies. When substance abuse by parents is one of the problems bringing children into the foster care system, multiple agency coordination is particularly important. Research suggests that a high percentage of children enter the foster care system because of parental substance abuse (Chipunga & Bent-Goodley, 2004). Neglect and physical abuse caused by parental substance abuse brought James into the foster care system and kept him in the system for many years.

When CPS removes a child from his or her parents' custody, a preferred placement option frequently is with a child's relatives. When there is an appropriate relative with whom to place a child, this arrangement may be satisfactory. It may provide an important family connection and stability for many children in out-of-home care. However, sometimes, the relative may be part of a multigenerational history of family abuse and neglect. This unfortunately was the case for James, as the case study will show. Nevertheless, his grandmother still was able to provide a home and some stability in his life for a period of time. However, after living with her for a number of years, her poor health and James' increasing aggressive behavior brought this placement option to an end. For a short time, he found some stability in a residential facility that was less than ideal, but kept him safe and he

The Systematic Mistreatment of Children in the Foster Care System
© 2007 by The Haworth Press, Taylor & Francis Group. All rights reserved.
doi:10.1300/5136_05

connected with a mental health therapist whom he trusted. After discharge from this facility, he then started down the road of entering and being quickly discharged from one placement after another, and sometimes living on the street. His health and well-being as well as his educational progress were severely compromised.

CASE STUDY OF JAMES

James, an African-American youth, lived with his mother and a younger and an older brother. James' mother's addiction to crack cocaine and alcohol made her unable, on an ongoing basis, to care for James and his two brothers. Her addiction led to her neglect of her children's physical and emotional needs. When she became angry, which was frequent at these times, she would hit James and his brothers with such force that they were left seriously bruised and otherwise injured.

Addiction and the physical abuse and neglect of children were not new in James' family. James' mother, as a child, experienced substantial physical abuse and neglect by her own mother (James' grandmother). When James' grandmother abused alcohol, she would hit his mother with anything she could get her hands on, leaving bruises and scars all over her body. During her bouts of drunkenness, she also failed to protect her daughter (James' mother) from sexual molestations. James' mother reported having been molested when she was eight and again when she was fourteen.

As an adult, James' mother was unable to maintain long-term relationships with men. Consequently, James and his brothers all had different fathers, none of whom were living with them when CPS became involved in their case. James had last seen his father when he was about two and did not remember him.

Alleged Physical Abuse and Neglect

When James was five and a half, a petition was filed with the juvenile court alleging that his mother, because of her addiction to drugs and alcohol, was unable to properly care for her children. Furthermore, she had inflicted numerous bruises and other injuries on James and his older brother and that such punishment was excessive and caused the children unreasonable pain and suffering. The petition stated that

James' father's whereabouts were unknown. The petition was sustained and James and his brothers were removed from their mother's custody.

Intervention

The CPS case plan for James and his brothers indicated that family reunification was the goal. James' mother was ordered to participate in a drug treatment program that included urine testing and psychiatric counseling.

Prevention

CPS placed James and his brothers in the home of their maternal grandmother when the petition was first filed, since it was the opinion of CPS that the boys were not safe when left in their mother's care. After the petition was sustained, the court ordered the children to remain with their grandmother despite the grandmother's record of abusing her own child, James' mother, when she was a child. Their mother was allowed to visit her children, but she was not allowed to be alone with them; her visits had to be monitored.

For the next three years, James and his brothers continued to live with their grandmother. James attended 87th Street School, the local elementary school in the neighborhood. School records from this period show James' reading skills to be below grade level and each year he seemed to become increasingly more disruptive in class (see Exhibit 5.1).

Advocacy Considerations

James and his brothers had a court-appointed lawyer at the time the petition was sustained and the court ordered the children to be placed with their grandmother in her home. A question that requires consideration is whether James and his brothers were well placed with their maternal grandmother and whether his lawyer should have raised this issue at the disposition hearing. This was a family with at least two generations of substance abuse leading to both physical abuse and neglect of the children. CPS, in the report to the court, noted the multigenerational substance abuse and domestic violence

EXHIBIT 5.1.
Placement History

Age	Placement	Maltreatment	School
5 yrs. 6 mos.	Grandmother	Neglect/ Abuse	87th St. Elem.
8 yrs. 10 mos.	Mother	Neglect/ Abuse	N/A
8 yrs. 11 mos.	Foster Home		N/A
9 yrs.	Grandmother		87th St. Elem/ NPS
10 yrs. 6 mos.	Martin Foster Home		Crestview NPS
10 yrs. 6 mos.	Mann Foster Home		Crestview NPS
10 yrs. 10 mos.	Psychiatric Hospital		Hospital School
11 yrs. 1 mo.	Grandmother		Crestview NPS
11 yrs. 2 mos.	Emergency Shelter		Shelter School
11 yrs 2 mos.	Grandmother		Crestview NPS
11 yrs. 2 mos.	Emergency Shelter		Shelter School
11 yrs. 3 mos.	Ford Group Home		Crestview NPS
11 yrs. 4 mos.	Highland Residential		On-grounds NPS
11 yrs. 4 mos.	Emergency Shelter		Shelter School
11 yrs. 7 mos.	Ford Group Home		Crestview NPS
11 yrs. 9 mos.	H & C Residential		On-grounds NPS
12 yrs. 5 mos.	Grandmother		N/A
12 yrs. 7 mos.	Gregory Group Home		Edgemont NPS
12 yrs. 8 mos.	Various Relatives		Edgemont NPS
12 yrs. 8 mos.	Various Relatives		Not in school
12 yrs. 11 mos.	Clayton Group Home		N/A
13 yrs.	Various Relatives		Not in school
13 yrs. 2 mos.	Emergency Shelter		Shelter School

Elem. = Elementary School.

N/A = No records available.

NPS = Nonpublic School (i.e., a private special education school).

in the family, but stressed instead the family strengths. These included, according to CPS:

- the grandmother's willingness to care for her daughter's children, making it possible for her to participate in an out-patient drug rehabilitation program,
- the grandmother's recognition of her own role in her daughter's problems, and
- the obvious love between the extended family members—specifically, the grandmother, James' mother, and James and his brothers.

Nevertheless, the undercurrent of domestic violence in the family remained a concern. During one of the visitations of James and his brothers by their mother, James' mother became involved in a physical altercation with James' grandmother as a result of an argument.

Intervention

Two years after the petition was filed, James' mother entered a residential drug rehabilitation program. She remained in the program for a year and made good progress. She completed a parenting course during that year and had plans to remain active in the post-graduation program, including attending, on a regular basis, meetings of Alcoholics Anonymous and Narcotics Anonymous. During his mother's stay in the drug rehabilitation program, she visited James and his brothers often, sometimes staying with them for up to twelve hours at the home of their grandmother. She was looking forward to having her children back and, as she came closer to completing her program, she had secured a full-time job as a staff assistant in a nursing home. She was going to start looking for housing near the nursing home and CPS recommended that her children be permitted a sixty-day visit with her as soon as she had obtained housing.

Extended Trial Placement with Their Mother

Two months before James turned nine, he and his brothers started living with their mother again. They had had some weekend visits with her in the apartment she had rented. Now, the boys were to remain with her for a sixty-day extended visit in preparation for their permanent reunification.

Less than a month into the sixty-day visit, the police were called to their mother's apartment with reports of domestic violence. When the police arrived, James and his older brother told them that their mother had left home with a male companion and had stayed away for two days. When their mother returned, James' older brother got into a physical fight with her that involved knives. The older brother ended up with some superficial cuts.

James' mother told the police that she had been drinking beer and smoking "primos" (a marijuana and cocaine combination). She also revealed that she had lost her job at the nursing home because she had failed to call and inform her supervisor of her absence. James and his brothers told the police that they did not want to remain with their mother.

What Had Gone Wrong?

Clearly, James' mother was not ready to live alone in the community and take on all the responsibilities that were required with a full-time job and three difficult boys. None of the boys had had any psychological counseling to help them deal with their feelings related to their mother's substance abuse.

Furthermore, it seems that James' mother needed a transitional setting, where she could have had the support of a drug rehabilitation program but, nonetheless, be able to have her sons living with her. In that type of supported context, they could learn to live together again and have a safety net to help them deal with the difficult issues that would arise. This type of program was not available for James' family.

Out-of-Home Placement

Prevention

The CPS social worker went into court immediately to change the placement order for James and his brothers. This court appearance was not a regularly scheduled placement review, but was put on what is called a "walk-on" calendar. The CPS recommendation was that the sixty-day extended visit be terminated and that the children be placed in a foster home. The reason for the foster home placement was that James' grandmother did not want to take her grandchildren back into her home because her own health was poor. Their grandmother had diabetes, high blood pressure, and generally poor health. Within a month, however, she reconsidered and requested that her grandsons be returned to her home. James and his brothers continued to live with their grandmother for another year and a half.

Minimum School Day

During this stay with his grandmother, James' behavioral problems at 87th Street School increased, causing him to be suspended from school frequently and put, for four months, on a minimum school-day schedule of three and a half hours per day. A physician who worked for the school district authorized the minimum day stating that it was required because James was "abusive to others—[he] leaves class and school without permission—[he gets into] fights—[and the] school police [had to be] called on multiple occasions."

At the time the school put James on a minimum school day, a referral for a special education assessment also was made. The referral stated that James' academic performance had deteriorated significantly in the previous five months, although it had been below grade level since the first grade. Furthermore, he needed constant supervision to complete any schoolwork and his attitude toward others had become increasingly hostile with frequent, seemingly unpredictable, aggressive outbursts, with both peers and adults. Also stated was that he was unable to accept adult authority and responded with hostility when corrected.

Four months after the referral for a special education assessment had been made and right before summer vacation, an individualized education program (IEP) meeting was held for James by his school district. The report from the assessment showed his cognitive ability to be in the average range and his academic achievement in reading was almost a year above his current fourth grade grade-level. He was about a year below grade-level in mathematics, and significantly below grade-level in his overall fund of knowledge. At the time, James was about three months shy of being ten years old, but his receptive language skills were judged to be at the five-year-old level. His assessment also showed deficits in auditory discrimination and short-term memory.

At the IEP meeting, James was found eligible for special education on the basis of having an emotional disturbance. The program that was recommended for him was a full-day special education class located at 87th Street School along with psychological counseling once a week. James started attending the special education program once school started in the fall, but his behavioral problems seemed to increase almost immediately. He cursed at his peers in this classroom. When he became angry, he threw chairs and turned over tables. He hit his peers frequently; at other times, he purposefully destroyed their clothing. He also left the classroom at will and would roam the campus.

James lasted only two months before another IEP meeting was held to change his school placement. The recommendation at this IEP meeting was for James to attend a nonpublic special education school. Also authorized was sixty minutes per week of psychological counseling. Within two weeks, James started attending Crestview School, a nonpublic school not far from his grandmother's house. James was in fifth grade at the time.

What Had Gone Wrong?

Prior to James becoming eligible for special education services, his school district used a medical exclusion to reduce his school day to three and a half hours. This was not an appropriate or a legally tenable way to change James' school program (Special Education Programs, 2005). What the school district should have done instead was to use the special education procedures in a more timely fashion. The school district made a referral for a special education assessment shortly after it reduced his school day. But the special education assessment timelines were greatly exceeded. Under state and federal law, a school district has sixty days to complete a special education assessment and return to an IEP meeting, but, in this case, James' district took 120 days (IDEA, 2004; Special Education Programs, 2005). The school district could have completed its assessment in just a few weeks and authorized special education services at that time, if it was really concerned about James' behavior in the general education classroom. In that way, he would not have been denied several hours per day of the compulsory education to which he was entitled. Instead, he could have been provided the support and structure he needed to function at school.

The school program that James' first IEP recommended did not provide the intensity of service that he required at that time. There is no information in the file about the capabilities of the classroom teacher, the behavior management system used in the classroom, or the number of students in the class and the types of emotional or behavioral problems that they had. But it seems clear that psychological counseling once a week for thirty minutes was not sufficient to deal with the array and intensity of behavioral problems James was exhibiting.

Another problem with the special education services provided for James was that no services were offered to address his receptive language and auditory discrimination problems identified in the school district's assessment. While James' emotional problems clearly were the priority in terms of providing him services, James' understanding of spoken language had been assessed as significantly delayed. He may have been misunderstanding what others said to him or what they meant by what they said.

Advocacy Considerations

When the time lines for James' assessment for special education were exceeded, his grandmother or other person involved in his life could have filed a special education noncompliance complaint with the state department of education or the federal Office for Civil rights to force the school district to comply with the law. Sometimes, just threatening to do this will encourage a negligent school to comply with the assessment timelines (see Exhibit 5.2).

EXHIBIT 5.2.
Filing a Noncompliance Complaint

When a school district violates a special education law, a parent or other person involved in a child's life may file a noncompliance complaint with the relevant state agency or the federal Office for Civil Rights (OCR). Filing a compliant consists of writing a letter describing the legal violation and providing evidence. The state agency or OCR then will investigate whether the district has violated a child's rights under federal or state special education law and, if so, require the district to engage in corrective action.

The school district should have recommended doing a functional behavioral assessment of James prior to recommending a change of school placement and, based on the findings, put together a behavioral implementation plan that would have become part of his IEP. A functional behavioral assessment is a detailed study of a child's behavior to determine the specific functions of a serious behavior problem— that is, how the misbehavior functions for him and how it serves a particular need.

Functional behavioral assessments involve reviewing a child's records, interviewing those who know the child well for clues about the behavior, and then doing extensive observations of the child at different times of the day and during different activities to understand when the behavior occurs, what precedes it, and what consequences follow it. State law (Hughes Bill, 1990), at the time, required that functional analysis assessments be done on any special education student who exhibited serious behavior problems, and whose behavior problems made it impossible for the student to achieve his IEP goals. James' behavior certainly satisfied these criteria (see Exhibit 5.3).

Placement in a Foster Home

Within a month of James' placement in Crestview nonpublic school, his grandmother decided that she no longer wanted to care for James and his brothers. The reason she gave for this decision, according to the court report, was because of James' mother's behavior toward her.

EXHIBIT 5.3.
Functional Behavioral Assessment

For special education students with serious behavior problems, request a functional behavioral assessment (sometimes called an functional analysis assessment) from the school district to determine under what circumstances the behaviors occur and what the student is getting from engaging in the behaviors (e.g., task avoidance, stimulation). Following a functional behavioral assessment, a behavioral intervention plan should be included in the student's IEP in order to help replace the student's negative behaviors with positive ones that fulfill the same function. (Assistance to States, 1997, §300.346)

She reported that the mother (her daughter) would enter her home un-invited, demand money, threaten and curse at her, take some of her possessions, and generally cause chaos. Because of the grandmother's poor health, she felt, that under these circumstances, she no longer could care for James and his brothers.

The boys, consequently, were placed in a foster home with foster parents Sadie and Joseph Martin, which was not to last very long. Seven days after the placement occurred, the foster father brought the boys into the CPS district office wanting them placed somewhere else. It was James' aggressive behavior and negative attitude that caused the foster father to request the change.

James and his brothers then were placed in a new foster home with foster mother Angela Mann. However, after a short period of time in this foster home, Angela requested that James be placed some-where else because of his aggressive, threatening, and angry behav-ior. Around this time, James' mother was incarcerated because of repeatedly having been picked up by the police for "driving under the influence."

Intervention

The social worker convinced Angela to keep James a while longer and authorized psychological therapy for him twice a week with a mental health professional. James, apparently not wanting to be re-moved from this foster home having started to form a relationship with the foster mother, agreed to the therapy sessions. In addition to attend-ing therapy with James and his brothers, Angela attended parenting classes authorized by CPS. It was not only James who was having se-rious behavior problems, but his brothers, not surprisingly, had started having them too.

Placement in a Psychiatric Hospital

James remained in the foster home with Angela Mann for five months before his behavior became so dangerous that CPS decided to have him admitted to a psychiatric hospital. He was ten years and ten months at the time.

James' foster mother described his continued dangerous behavior during the four months with this foster family as including: frequent physical fights, striking others seemingly without provocation, throwing furniture, and threatening to kill them. Many of these behaviors also had been reported in the school setting. In some instances, James was so aggressive toward his peers that he had to be physically restrained by adults, and the peers whom he attacked required medical attention.

Intervention

James initially was put on a "seventy-two-hour hold" (Lanterman-Petris-Short [LPS] Act, 1968) in the hospital because, during an intake interview, he was assessed as being a danger to others and, therefore, not safe to remain in the community. Once the seventy-two-hour hold was up, the hospital mental health staff determined that James still was a danger to others and extended the hold to fourteen days.

During this period of time, the mental health director and psychiatric social worker at the hospital wrote a letter to the judge of the juvenile court requesting a voluntary court order to cover ongoing inpatient mental health treatment for James that included behavioral interventions and medication. They estimated the length of inpatient treatment that James needed to be between two and four months. A court hearing was held and James agreed to the voluntary placement at the psychiatric hospital.

The hospital's psychiatristic admitting report noted that James' responses when asked what his three wishes were, at the time, all related to his mother. These wishes indicate how strongly he was affected by his separation from his mother and the problems in her life. He wished: (1) to be with my mother; (2) for my mother to stop drinking; and (3) for my mother to be out of jail.

James' hospital treatment consisted of milieu, individual, family, recreational, and group therapy. In addition, he attended the hospital school. His program was supplemented with medication. He was taking Tegretol, a seizure medication, to decrease his anger and irritability and, in the first months of his stay at the hospital, Haldol, an antipsychotic medication to reduce his agitation.

James seemed to respond well to his regimen at the hospital. The records indicate that at a certain point, he realized he had to behave well in order to leave the hospital and this realization led to his significantly changed behavior. He began to earn the highest behavioral rating (indicating high compliance with behavioral expectations) for his behavior on the living unit. During James' ten-week stay at the hospital, his behavior improved remarkably. Nevertheless, his discharge diagnosis was Conduct Disorder, solitary aggressive type. He also was described as having a "chronic mixed emotional and behavioral syndrome . . . [t]he feelings most prominent include[d] anger/resentment, sadness, anxiety/fear, blaming, guilt, and shame/humiliation."

Aggressive Behavior Leading to Placement Instability

While James was hospitalized, Advocacy Services senior attorney, Nancy Shea, was appointed to represent him. The purpose of this representation was to help identify an appropriate living situation for James, thus stabilizing his placement.

James then was discharged from the hospital to the care of his grandmother. Follow-up outpatient psychiatric care was slated to continue at the mental health clinic connected to the hospital. James returned to Crestview, the nonpublic school he previously had attended.

Unfortunately, James' grandmother failed to attend many of the weekly therapy sessions at the mental health clinic scheduled for her and James. She claimed her absences were due to her poor health. Within a month of James' discharge from the hospital, James' grandmother no longer felt she could handle him and he was removed from her home and sent to the county emergency shelter. James presumably had become physically aggressive with his grandmother, threatening her with a knife. Several days after James was sent to the emergency shelter, his grandmother started feeling guilty about having sent him away and requested that he be returned to her care, which he was. However, he again became physically aggressive at her home, destroying property and physically threatening family members. So his grandmother requested his removal and James once again was returned to the emergency shelter.

Within a month, he was placed in the Ford Group Home pending his acceptance at Highland Residential Treatment Center, a facility that Nancy had recommended as a preferred placement option for James, that is if the clinical staff would accept him. Highland was considered one of the best residential treatment programs in the county. But this facility did not typically accept youngsters who had a high propensity for physical aggression and this was the only reservation that Advocacy Services staff had.

Somewhat surprisingly, Highland Residential accepted James and a month later, he was placed in their most restrictive and highly therapeutic cottage. Unfortunately, he lasted there only one week before the staff insisted on his removal from the facility. They were concerned about the safety of the facility staff and residents based on the behavior they had seen from James that week. James had assaulted staff and peers and was completely uncooperative with the facility psychiatrist, refusing all medication. He also refused to attend school. Consequently, James was removed from this facility and returned to the emergency shelter.

What Had Gone Wrong?

The structure that the hospital program provided for James had worked to contain his physical and verbal aggressive behavior. He was motivated to follow the program so as to bring about his discharge. Placement at his grandmother's home clearly did not provide the structure and level of service intensity that he needed. The fact that James' grandmother missed many of their outpatient therapy sessions seems likely to have contributed to the quick demise of James' placement with her.

For a youngster like James, placement at his grandmother's might have worked upon discharge from the hospital if, initially, more mental health services could have been provided to the family on a daily basis in the home. These daily services would have monitored James' compliance with taking his medication and also would have helped James and his grandmother work out any problems between them in a constructive, nonphysical way. A reward system for James' compliance with set behavioral goals could have been put in place and maintained by an in-home, itinerant, mental health professional. Crisis intervention services also would have been important as a component to this in-home package of services.

With the quick demise of James' placement with his grandmother, he seemed to continue in his downward spiral of physical aggression as his way of dealing with a world that he would have preferred had other choices for him. He did not have the option of living with his mother, who, when released from jail, was stuck in a substance abusing, unstable lifestyle. She did not have a permanent place to live and, while she would tell the CPS social worker that she intended to enroll in another drug rehabilitation treatment facility, she did not enroll at this time. She kept in touch with her children, but her inability to get her life together must have been difficult for James and brought up emotions that he was ill equipped to resolve.

Return to the Emergency Shelter

James was eleven years and four months when he returned to the emergency shelter. He remained there for three months. He, not unlike other difficult children placed there, seemed to do fairly well. The emergency shelter was a place that his social worker described as having limited expectations for the youngsters there and providing them with frequent rewards.

I met with James while he was at the emergency shelter. James, at first, did not look at me and just hung his head. He seemed depressed and was uncommunicative, but appeared to listen to what I had to say. I let him know that I worked with his attorney and that it was my responsibility to try to get him appropriate educational services.

Within a month of James' return to the emergency shelter, a legally required IEP meeting was held for him (Special Education Programs, 2005). Based on the recommendation of the teacher and administrator from the emergency shelter school, his classroom placement was to be a full-day special education class, psychological counseling once a week for twenty to thirty minutes, and forty-five minutes per week of the services of a behavior management aide. He also was to be referred for an assessment to determine his need for speech and language services.

A Referral to the Department of Mental Health

James was eleven years and seven months when he entered the Ford Group Home this time. He remained there for just over two months. This particular group home was part of a small network of group homes owned by the same person. In order to try to preserve James' placement in this group home network, the owner moved James from one home to another and spent considerable time with him trying to help him adjust and to decrease his aggressive behavior. Nevertheless, James' behavior proved to be too difficult and he again was discharged from this placement.

While living at the Ford Group Home, however, James had reentered Crestview, the nonpublic school he previously attended, although now he was at the junior high campus. An IEP meeting was held within thirty days of James' placement at Crestview and I attended the meeting. The explicit purpose of this meeting was to initiate a referral to DMH for James. All members of this IEP team easily agreed to the DMH referral. The school district also had to authorize the funding for the nonpublic school he was attending, which it did. The school district promptly followed through with the DMH referral shortly after the meeting.

I made arrangements to observe James at Crestview, but when I showed up on the date scheduled, the administrator at the school told me that James had been terminated from the program, the reason, of course, being his aggressive behavior. I also learned that he no longer resided in the group home either, and had been moved to a residential treatment facility in another part of the city.

What Had Gone Wrong?

I, of course, was annoyed that no one from the school called to inform me that James had been thrown out of the nonpublic school in light of the fact that I had a scheduled appointment. Nor had our office been informed that James was now in a different living situation as well. However, knowing the seriousness of his behavior problems, I suppose I should have called ahead that morning to check if James was still in attendance at the school.

A Residential Treatment Facility

Intervention

James' next placement was at a large residential treatment facility, called H & C Residential, with an on-grounds nonpublic school. This facility primarily housed adolescent boys from the delinquency system, placed there by the probation department. The program provided individual psychological therapy once a week on a regular basis, and up to three times a week if needed. There also was group therapy five times a week and medication consultation and monitoring by a psychiatrist. James was eleven years and nine months at the time of placement and the youngest boy at the facility.

Soon after I learned that James had been placed at H & C Residential Treatment Center, I contacted DMH to inform the coordinator of the assessment unit that James' placement had changed. I was fairly certain that no one else would transmit this information. The assessment coordinator indicated that James' case would have to be transferred to a different assessment unit in the county, one that was responsible for the area in which his new residential facility was located. I then called the coordinator of the assessment unit to which James' case was being transferred to inform her that James' case was on the way to her unit and to please be on the lookout for it. She and I had worked together on many cases and had a good working relationship. She agreed to have the DMH evaluation of James done promptly and to attend the IEP that would follow the evaluation.

I called the school attached to this residential treatment facility to make arrangements to observe James in his classroom and meet with the school administrator and his therapist. Once at the school, I was not very impressed, to say the least, about what I observed in the classroom. James had his head down on the desk during the entire class. The teacher informed me that what I was seeing was a fairly typical picture of how James functioned on most days. She did not seem to have much insight into why James was not participating in class.

From my observation of the work that the class was doing and the comments of the other students, it was quite obvious that James' intellectual ability was at a much higher level than the other students in the class. Another concern I had was that the teacher was new and, more importantly, had no special education credential or training.

My meeting with the administrator of the school was equally disappointing. She did not have an education background and seemed to know little about improving learning for youngsters who had the kinds of problems James had. She was not aware that James was not participating in class and could not tell me why he was placed in a classroom with students who were much lower cognitively functioning than he was.

I was impressed, however, with James' therapist. He seemed, in a short period of time, to have formed a therapeutic relationship with James and had a good understanding of the psychological issues negatively affecting James' behavior. He too was unaware, however, that James kept his head on his desk most of the time in class. The therapist told me that James currently was experiencing a significant amount of depression, but he would have the treating psychiatrist monitor his medication more closely.

Advocacy Considerations

When James moved from the group home to the residential treatment facility, I knew there was a high likelihood that his DMH referral could be stalled. I knew if I did not take the initiative and inform the DMH assessment coordinators of James' change of placement it most likely would take some time before they knew about it. I wanted to make sure that nothing happened to derail the assessment process. It was helpful in that when James moved from the Ford Group Home to H & C Residential, he remained in the same school district. As a result, a new referral to DMH was not required. In addition, the fact that I knew the assessment coordinators from other cases on which I had worked and had a particularly good relationship with one helped move the case forward and keep it on track (see Exhibit 5.4).

Department of Mental Health Assessment and School Observations

The DMH assessment coordinator called and informed me that the evaluator had completed the mental health evaluation of James. I told

---

EXHIBIT 5.4.
The Role of Those Representing the Child

Those representing a foster youth frequently must play the role of the youth's case carrier in order to increase the chances that referrals are made and services received.

the assessment coordinator that I would contact the school district currently responsible for James to set up an IEP meeting. I called the school district administrator responsible for setting up IEP meetings for children residing in James' residential treatment facility and an IEP meeting for James was scheduled soon after.

Before the IEP meeting, I went to observe James in his school placement again. I wanted to see if James had started participating in class. I made arrangement to visit the school on a particular day and time, but when I arrived, I learned that James had been taken to see a dentist and, consequently, he was not there. I also learned he had been placed in another classroom, so, rather than not accomplishing anything on this trip to the facility, I spent a little time meeting with the teacher. James' classroom was comprised of youngsters who were several years older than he was. I also learned the classroom teacher had no teaching credential from our state, had taught physical education in another state, and had no special education training.

I returned to the school on another occasion and did get to observe James in his new classroom this time. He was somewhat disruptive and not very involved in the class activity, but at least he was not sleeping through this class with his head on the desk.

Advocacy Considerations

I obviously had forgotten the lesson I should have learned from my previous attempt to observe James at school. For many children in the foster care system, even with a scheduled appointment, it is important to call ahead the morning of a classroom observation to ascertain if the child is still in attendance at the school and is actually in the class (see Exhibit 5.5).

EXHIBIT 5.5.
Arrangements for School Observations

When going to observe a youth in his or her class at school, it is a good idea to check with the school on the morning of the visit to make sure the youth is still in attendance at the school and is at school that day.

IEP Meeting to Review DMH Assessment

I attended James' IEP meeting as his representative from our office. When I walked in to the meeting, most of the other members of the team were already present, including James. The CPS worker seemed unclear as to who I was and James quickly said, "She's here for me." I was touched by the way he said this and felt that I had made a connection with him. I let James and the IEP team members know that it was not necessary that James attend the entire meeting, unless he chose to. I explained to James what would be covered in the meeting. He seemed relieved not to have to be part of the entire meeting and decided to go back to the unit before the DMH assessment of him was discussed.

The coordinator of the DMH assessment unit shared her agency's evaluation of James. She let us know that she had handpicked the evaluator who evaluated James. He was an African-American man who was a Licensed Clinical Social Worker and had a knack for communicating well with aggressive, oppositional youngsters like James.

The DMH assessment consisted of a review of James' school, psychological, and psychiatric records, a clinical interview with him, and interviews with his grandmother and his current therapist and teacher. The assessment report described James as having "feelings of rejection and abandonment by [his] mother and father [that] appeared to have intensified recently when his grandmother and legal guardian had him placed out of home, because he was a severe behavioral problem and beyond her control." The report went on to say that James was "evidencing severe behavioral problems including hostile, angry, aggressive behavior, explosive episodes, noncompliant and oppositional behavior and defiant, extremely verbally abusive and disrespectful behavior toward authority figures." James also was manifesting "a chronic mild depression which appears to have deepened recently triggered by a resurfacing of aforementioned abandonment issues." The report continued by describing James as having "fragile defense mechanisms [that] are primarily avoidance and denial of issues and feelings giving way to acting out behavior as a means to fend off the depression." The evaluator noted that James appeared to be "a youth of bright normal intelligence with the potential to be successful in school if behavioral and emotional problems could be ameliorated."

The report concluded that the appropriate educational setting for James was a nonpublic school, and to meet his psychological needs, he required individual and family counseling/therapy along with medication evaluation and monitoring.

James already was receiving individual and group therapy services from the residential treatment facility, and, at the meeting, the therapist agreed to initiate family therapy sessions with both James and his grandmother. At my request, DMH agreed to provide ongoing case management services for James in order to monitor his overall mental health treatment needs. As part of the case management services, the DMH coordinator recommended that the IEP team reconvene in ninety days and, at that time, determine whether James had additional mental health needs that were not being properly addressed.

James' therapist then reported that James had verbalized to him the very real problems he had in trusting others. He also had communicated to his therapist his feelings of depression that strongly emerged the previous week related to his brother having a birthday and James not being able to be with him. As a consequence of James' depression and subsequent acting out with angry, aggressive behavior, the therapist reported that James lost his privilege of spending the weekend at his grandmother's home. This led to James having feelings of hopelessness and that nothing else really mattered.

Several of the IEP team members expressed concern that James was the youngest resident at this treatment facility and that the boys there primarily were placed by the probation department. However, his CPS social worker acknowledged that group homes had not been successful at dealing with James' problems and his options for placement were fairly limited. Nevertheless, James' CPS social worker agreed to work with the DMH placement unit when James was either ready to leave this residential treatment facility or if he simply needed another placement because of not doing well in the current placement. The school district administrator agreed to work with both CPS and DMH to identify an appropriate nonpublic school placement for James when a change of placement was imminent.

I also requested that James be assessed to determine if he had a specific learning disability in the area of understanding language. There had been evidence of that in a previous assessment and I wanted clarity on the issue. The school district said that the nonpublic school at H & C Residential had the responsibility of doing this assessment, since it was a covered expense in the contract that the district had with the nonpublic school. The nonpublic school administrator agreed to evaluate James for an expressive-language-related learning disability.

I left the meeting feeling pleased that I had made some headway in getting the different agencies responsible for James to work together, hopefully, to his benefit. I also felt it was time to have more assessment information about whether James had problems related to understanding spoken language and, if so, were they connected in any way to his behavioral problems.

Advocacy Considerations

One of my goals at this IEP meeting was to try to get the school district, DMH, and CPS to work together. So that when James was going to be moved to a new placement, the choice of where he would move would benefit from the expertise of the three agencies responsible for him. DMH had serious concerns about the residential treatment facility where CPS had placed him, since it was a facility where he was the youngest resident and there were few others in his age range. Furthermore, it was a facility housing primarily delinquent older adolescent males. DMH had considerable expertise in appropriately matching youngsters with mental health needs to the available residential treatment facilities. But, CPS had not called on DMH for assistance in this area prior to placing him in this particular residential treatment facility.

The administrator from the school district had expertise in matching youngsters having emotional and behavioral problems to appropriate nonpublic schools in the city. This administrator did not think much of the on-grounds nonpublic school at James' current residential facility. He had observed the program many times and had spoken with the administrator and he had felt the educational program was extremely weak.

I believed that if the three agencies—CPS, DMH, and the school district—would work together prior to a placement change for James, then the likelihood of an appropriate placement for him would be increased.

IEP Review Meeting

In slightly less than ninety days, another IEP meeting was held. This meeting was specifically to discuss future placements for James and to see how he was faring in his current placement. Just prior to the meeting, I learned that James' case had been transferred to a new CPS social worker. I contacted her and informed her about the IEP meeting. She planned to attend, but, at the last minute, had to go to court on another case. Consequently, the IEP team was unable to discuss future placement options without the input of James' CPS social worker.

The nonpublic school presented its evaluation of James, but it was done so poorly that it did not give the IEP team the information it needed to determine if James had an expressive-language-related learning disability. Rather than have the nonpublic school do further evaluation, the school district agreed to do it. The school district realized it would be futile to have the nonpublic school do additional evaluation in this area.

We learned at this meeting that James had made some progress in his residential program during the past three months. He also had several successful home visits with his grandmother.

What Had Gone Wrong?

James' CPS case had to be transferred to a new social worker since the one he had was no longer working for CPS. The previous worker, before leaving the agency, failed to brief his supervisor about the coordination efforts between the agencies that had been agreed with regards to selecting the next placement for James. Consequently, when a new social worker was appointed, she was not told about the commitment of the agencies to work together on James' behalf and why this was so needed in this case. I tried to brief her in this area, but I was not sure she really understood why the coordination was so important. The problems that followed might have been averted, had the interagency coordination worked better.

Placement with Grandmother

Over the winter vacation, James was released from the residential facility to the care of his grandmother. CPS and the residential facility arranged this change of placement without contacting Advocacy Services, DMH, or the school district. As a result, there were no mental health services set up for James and his grandmother and a school placement had not been identified.

We, at Advocacy Services, learned that James no longer was residing at the residential treatment facility when we received a phone call from his aunt. She wanted us to help arrange a school placement for him. Since it was winter break, the schools were closed and we really could not do anything until they reopened in the beginning of January.

I talked with James and he told me that he wanted to attend the local public middle school. I was concerned that he would not be successful in a large public school setting and shared my concerns with him, but he still wanted to try the middle school, so I decided to see whether we could make it work.

I observed the special education special day class at the school and liked the teacher. Even though the school was quite large, the special education class was small. When I told the teacher about James, she felt that she would be able to handle him. I arranged with a school district administrator with whom I had worked closely on many cases to allow James to enroll in this school, although his IEP still indicated nonpublic school placement. The administrator told me we would have a new IEP meeting once James started at the school.

The next day James and his adult cousin went to the middle school to enroll James. While James was filling out the school forms, the assistant principal noticed he was using a style of block-like printing associated with gangs. The assistant principal told James to stop using that type of printing. James refused to change the way he was writing and, instead, left the school angry, never to return.

What Had Gone Wrong?

James was discharged from the residential treatment facility over the winter break. While it surely was nice for James that he was able to be with his relatives for the holidays, it was a terrible time to try to get services in place for him. The schools were closed and the mental health clinics were operating with reduced staffs. James' CPS social worker did James a disservice to allow him to be discharged from the residential facility at this time of the year without school and mental health services in place.

Advocacy Considerations

Since James had an IEP that specified nonpublic school as the appropriate placement, when he was placed back with his grandmother, he should have been enrolled in a nonpublic school close to her home. When James wanted to attend the local public middle school, an IEP meeting should have been held beforehand to bring about this school placement change. The reason, in this case, it did not occur that way was that James was out of school and it would have taken some time to put the IEP team together. We wanted James back in school as soon as possible. Consequently, the district administrator called the assistant principal at the middle school and requested that he enroll James using his current IEP and that an IEP meeting would soon be convened once James started in this setting. As it happened, there was no need to change James' IEP because he never started at the middle school.

Group Home Placement

Without mental health services and a school placement for James in place, James' behavior quickly deteriorated and within two months, his grandmother could not handle him. His grandmother was quite ill. James, however, was refusing to be placed in another group home and was living on the streets. At the request of his aunt, the police picked him up. CPS was notified and James was placed in the Gregory Group Home, near where his grandmother lived.

I recommended Edgemont nonpublic school for James since it was not far from his group home and the school would transport him from home to school and back again. James' CPS worker agreed to meet me at Edgemont to observe how the program functioned and to talk with its administrator before deciding to enroll James there. We both felt this nonpublic school could work with James and it had a somewhat decent academic program, which was a significant improvement from the nonpublic school at H & C Residential he had attended. James' social worker brought him to Edgemont School a day or two later to be interviewed by the school administrator. We felt a sigh of relief when James and the administrator hit it off and James was enrolled in this school.

Several weeks after James started attending Edgemont School, he abruptly was discharged from the Gregory Group Home for violating the rules. He then was placed back in the home of his grandmother. However, because of her ill health and inability to care for him he started moving from the home of one relative to another.

Back with Relatives Again

James continued attending Edgemont School as he moved between the homes of his relatives. He continued there for close to two more months before he was expelled for trying to buy a gun from another student.

At this point, James was becoming more and more difficult to deal with and out of control of his relatives. I talked with his cousin on several occasions, but it was not clear where James actually was living and his relatives seemed incapable of supervising him. He was out of school and had no school to attend. I set up an appointment for James to be interviewed by another nonpublic school, one that had a reputation of working well with youngsters with extremely difficult behavior. A medical appointment also was arranged for James because his CPS worker was concerned that he had not seen a medical doctor for quite some time and was in need of medication to help control his behavior. James' cousin was aware of both appointments and told us she definitely would get James to the appointments, but neither she nor James showed up at either appointment. It became clear that James' relatives not only had no control over him, but also did not even know where he was most of the time.

We, at Advocacy Services, had serious concerns and wanted James' CPS social worker to intercede. We were fairly certain that James had become involved with a local gang. We wanted his social worker to place him at the emergency shelter because he would be safe there and off the streets.

To our surprise, James' social worker said that she was unable to place children at the emergency shelter anymore, if there were any other placements in the county that would take them. She said it did not matter whether the available placements were ones from which the children were likely to run away. The social worker also reported that she had sent a packet of information about James to Moontree, the residential treatment facility where Sharon had been placed when I first met her. This was the only facility in the county that had a locked unit. James' cousin had agreed to care for James, in the interim, if he was in school, but, at the moment, no one seemed to know where he was.

James again was picked up by the police, but fairly quickly re-leased to the parents of a friend of his. He then returned to his aunt's house and she agreed to keep him until he was placed in a residential facility. Interviews were scheduled at another nonpublic school; how-ever, he and his aunt never showed up for their interviews. Neither did they show up for another medical appointment that had been sched-uled for James. We contacted the CPS social worker and she told us that James now ran away each time an appointment was scheduled for him.

Several days later, James showed up at his aunt's house. She wanted him removed immediately. James' social worker found him a placement at Clayton Group Home in another part of the city, far from where his relatives lived, and took James there. We still wanted him placed at the emergency shelter. The social worker told us she had no choice in the matter.

I had a conversation with one of the staff at the Clayton Group Home and let this person know that James was a runaway risk. This staff member told me they had experience dealing with youngsters like James, but there was only so much they could do because their facility was not locked. Not unexpectedly, James ran away from the group home and ended up back at his aunt's house. She decided to let him stay because, she told us, she wanted to keep the family together. Her goal was to get him in school and on medication. Doctors' ap-pointments were made and an interview was scheduled at a nonpublic school. But again, not unexpectedly, James and his aunt never made it to any of the appointments because James always would disappear at those times. A couple of day's later, James ended up at his grand-mother's house, and she decided he could stay with her for a short period of time.

James' CPS social worker made an appointment for him to be in-terviewed by Moontree Residential Treatment. This was the facility with a locked unit. James actually went with his social worker to the interview. The social worker told us that there would be an opening at this facility in three weeks. At the interview, however, James told the administrator that he did not want to be placed at Moontree. His social worker tried to talk him into considering this placement and James reluctantly agreed that he would.

One of James' aunts agreed that James could live with her for the next three weeks. A little over a week later, however, the aunt decided that James could no longer stay at her home. Nancy told his social worker that she wanted James in the emergency shelter. The social worker again reiterated that she could not place him there. James' aunt then decided to take things into her own hands and called the police and had James picked up and taken to the emergency shelter.

Once at the emergency shelter, James called Nancy and told her that he wanted to go back to his family. Nancy let James know that she would not make arrangements to send him back to his relatives. He called back two days later and told her that one of his aunts had agreed to take him in. Nancy again told James she would not agree to that arrangement for him.

Under the circumstances, James' social worker now was resigned to keep James at the emergency shelter for the time being and ordered medical evaluations for him there. She also warned the emergency shelter staff that James was a runaway risk. But the information that stunned us was that the social worker reported that James' mother finally has entered another drug rehabilitation program and the social worker was hopeful the family might be able to reunify soon.

What Had Gone Wrong?

Why was James' social worker unable to send him to the county emergency shelter when he seemed to be living on the streets and his relatives had no control over him? At that time, CPS was trying to keep foster children from continually returning to the emergency shelter and to stop children from long-term placements there. The purpose was to try to provide foster youth with permanent placements in the community as child welfare law required and to save the county the high cost of placement when children remained at the emergency shelter for longer than thirty days. The problem with this policy, however, was the CPS social worker was rendered impotent in the face of a youngster like James. She certainly was not fulfilling her responsibility to keep him safe.

Advocacy Considerations

Why did Advocacy Services not go into the juvenile court and ask the judge to order James picked up and placed in the emergency shelter? Nancy's concern was that the judge in the particular courtroom in which James' case was heard was not easy to work with and had little tolerance for youth like James. Her fear was that the judge would change James' status from a dependent to a delinquent, which likely would land him in juvenile hall or the youth authority. We still believed there were residential placement options within the dependency system that could address James' needs better than those in the delinquency system.

CONCLUSION

I often wonder how things might have turned out for James if he had been able to live with his mother and brothers in a facility that would have provided his mother with the support and structure she needed to abstain from abusing drugs and alcohol. For children like James, and others who end up in the foster care system because of parental substance abuse, there is a need for a supported-living placement option for families that could not stay together otherwise. James suffered considerably from his feelings of abandonment by his mother. His anger and aggressive behavior only increased as he moved into adolescence. Keeping such a family together in a supported living environment with ongoing psychological therapy and appropriate substance abuse support groups would appear to make much more sense and create stability and security for children rather than the kind of placement history that James endured.

SUMMARY

The purpose of this chapter was to show how the placement options available to James were not adequate to meet his needs and there was no existing placement option that would have allowed him and his brothers to live successfully with their mother. While being placed with his grandmother, they never received the type of intensive in-home services that might have made foster care placement with her viable on a long-term basis. Furthermore, CPS did not ensure that school and mental health services were in place when James was discharged from a residential treatment facility.

Chapter 6

Silvia and Carlos:
Placing Siblings Together
in a Foster Home

INTRODUCTION

As in James' case, parental substance abuse by Silvia and Carlos' parents led to neglect and physical abuse of the children. A petition alleging parental neglect was filed before the adjudication hearing. Then child protective services (CPS) commissioned the services of a psychologist to help determine the appropriate course of action to take with the children. CPS also developed a case plan that required the parents to seek help for their alcohol abuse, among other requirements, in order to maintain custody of their children. However, when the parents failed to follow through with the requirements of the case plan, the children were removed from their home.

Once removed from their parents, Silvia remained with one foster family during her entire out-of-home placement experience. Carlos, however, did not have such a stable placement history. CPS, on the recommendation of the psychological assessment, placed each child, as well as another sibling, in separate foster or group home placements.

An important question that Silvia and Carlos' case raises is whether siblings should be placed in the same foster or group home when entering and continuing to stay in the foster care system? CPS must make this determination and those who represent foster children also must determine what constitutes the best interests of the children in this important area.

The Systematic Mistreatment of Children in the Foster Care System
© 2007 by The Haworth Press, Taylor & Francis Group. All rights reserved.
doi:10.1300/5136_06

115

There are no national figures of how many children in foster care have siblings or how many were placed with their siblings when they entered foster care. Two states, California and New York, which account for a large number of children in out-of-home care, however, do collect sibling placement data. In 2002, of the 91,509 children who were in county supervised foster care in California, 71 percent of these children had at least one sibling in out-of-home care. Forty percent of these children were placed with all of their siblings who were also in out-of-home care. However, about 42 percent of the total number of children in foster care in the state—or 38,657 children—were separated from one or more of their siblings (Casey Family Programs, 2003).

Data from New York City also present a similar picture. Of the 11,215 children who entered foster care in 1999, 66.9 percent had siblings also in out-of-home care. Of these, 47 percent, or 3,525 children were separated from at least one of their siblings. That represents nearly one-third of all the children who entered out-of-home care in the city that year (Casey Family Programs, 2003).

The most common reason that siblings are separated in foster care is logistical. Foster homes that are licensed to care for multiple children may fill up in a piecemeal fashion (Lawrence & Lankford, 1997). For example, a foster parent who is licensed to care for six children may be sent two children from one family, three children from three different families, and then have only one opening for another child. In this case, the foster parent would not have room for two siblings from a family that recently entered the foster care system and needed placement.

Other common reasons for which siblings have been separated are to provide individual attention to each child, to prevent an older child from continuing to play a parental role, to prevent sibling rivalry, or to provide specialized care to children with special needs. The Casey Family Programs (2003) refers to these reasons as "sibling placement myths" that lack a factual basis.

CASE STUDY OF SILVIA AND CARLOS

Silvia was born in Guatemala and Carlos in the United States. Their parents, Mariana and Arnulfo, had come to the United States when

Silvia and her sister, Ana, who had mild autism and mild mental retardation, were of preschool age. Mariana and the children arrived first and lived with relatives in the United States. But within a year, through working and borrowing money, Mariana was able to send money to her husband so he too could join her.

Arnulfo arrived in the United States and the family initially continued to live with relatives. Arnulfo then found work in a factory. Carlos was born around this time and the family moved to an apartment. Several years after Carlos' birth, the factory closed down and, consequently, Arnulfo lost his job. Unable to find a new job, Arnulfo started collecting bottles and cans on the street, enabling him to bring home $5 to $10 a day and help put "milk on the table." Unfortunately, the money was not all spent on milk. About this time, Mariana started drinking heavily.

Suspected Child Abuse

When Ana was seventeen, her teacher filed a child abuse report because Ana reported that her mother had beaten her with a belt. When CPS did its investigation, the investigating social worker found the conditions of the family's home to be "filthy and unsanitary," including rotting food on the stove and in the refrigerator, a lack of edible food in the house, and dirty bedrooms with mice running under the beds and through the piles of clothing on the floor. The parents, according to the social worker, drank on a daily basis, with Mariana in particular becoming severely intoxicated. Day-to-day life for the children was very chaotic. The children reported to the CPS worker that their parents frequently yelled at them, and their mother hit them with whatever object she had close to her. The parents also argued with each other, which lead to yelling matches and physical altercations. In addition, the children rarely went to school and Mariana insisted they stay at home and often told them they were "sick."

The Petition

CPS filed a petition with the juvenile court alleging that the children's parents were frequent users of alcohol, and that the alcohol use limited their ability to provide regular care for their children. In addition, the petition stated that on various occasions the mother inflicted welts and other bruises on the children's bodies using her hand or objects such as a belt, a cord, or a broom. Furthermore, the parents failed to provide their children with the basic necessities of life such as edible food; a safe, clean home; clean clothing; medical care; and an education.

Intervention

Prior to the adjudication hearing, the CPS social worker who was assigned to the case tried to work with the parents to alleviate the problems enumerated in the juvenile court petition. The social worker set forth, in a service plan, tasks on which the parents were required to follow through. These included cleaning up the house, sending the children to school, and obtaining help for their alcohol abuse.

Prevention

When the parents failed to follow through on these tasks and continued drinking to the point of inebriation, the social worker detained the children and took them into protective custody, thus removing them from their parents' home. CPS placed Silvia and Carlos in separate foster homes and Ana in a small group home until the adjudication hearing. Ana was seventeen, Silvia sixteen, and Carlos was nine when the children were removed from their parents' home.

Adjudication/Disposition

Prior to the adjudication hearing, the court ordered a psychological evaluation of the three children and the parents in order to obtain expert opinion on the following questions: (1) the likelihood of the children being physically abused if returned home; (2) the extent of the parents' substance abuse and its effect on the children; (3) the type of relationship that existed between the parents and the children; and (4) specific recommendations for placement and custody of the children, visitation of the children by the parents, plans for reunification of the family, and the need for psychological therapy for the family members.

After separate clinical interviews with each child and parent and the administration of psychological testing, the psychologist came to some serious conclusions. It was his opinion that the damage to the children, as a result of their parents' alcoholism, was already severe.

The parents were in denial of their alcoholism, were extremely dysfunctional, and had deteriorated recently in their ability to care for their children. The psychologist recommended that the children remain placed out of the home and in separate foster homes to ensure they would each receive individual attention. He recommended that each of the children receive educational interventions, since they were functioning below their potential in school. He also recommended that they attend summer school. Ana had had an individualized education program (IEP) since the second grade, based on her mild autism and mental retardation, but he recommended that Silvia and Carlos receive an evaluation to determine if they had disabilities that would qualify them for special education services. He also indicated that the children would benefit from counseling to address their emotional difficulties, which were related to the dysfunctional family environment in which they had lived. The only contact he recommended that the parents have with their children should be monitored at the CPS office. The reason for this recommendation was that Mariana had been intoxicated when she visited Silvia in her foster home and had had a phone conversation with Carlos, presumably while intoxicated, and had upset him significantly by her inappropriate remarks.

At the adjudication hearing, the petition was sustained. The court ordered that the children be suitably placed. The parents were ordered by the court to participate in an alcohol abuse program with random testing, parenting classes, and individual counseling. They were allowed one visit per week at the children's places of residence, but it had to be monitored and they would not be allowed to visit their children if they were intoxicated (see Exhibits 6.1 and 6.2).

EXHIBIT 6.1.
Silvia's Placement History

Age	Placement	Maltreatment	School
16 yrs.	Gonzalez Foster Home	Neglect/Abuse	Rogers H.S.
18 1/3 yrs.	Gonzalez Foster Home		Cleveland H.S.

H.S. = High School.

EXHIBIT 6.2.
Carlos' Placement History

Age	Placement	Maltreatment	School
9 yrs. 3 mos.	Foster Home	Neglect/Abuse	Sunnyslope Elem.
9 yrs. 11 mos.	Relatives		57th St. Elem.
10 yrs 4 mos.	Foster Home		Euclid Elem.
11 yrs.1 mo.	Gonzalez Foster Home		Oak St. Elem.

Elem. = Elementary School.

Ana and Her Parents' Disappearance

The children remained in the homes in which they originally had been placed. Ana was very unhappy in the Harris Group Home and complained that Martha Ortiz, the house parent, mistreated her and that the other girls in the home made fun of her. One afternoon, Ana left the group home by herself and never returned. CPS learned through Silvia and Carlos, who had spoken to their parents by phone that they had arranged to pick up Ana once she left the group home. This apparently is what happened. Mariana, Arnulfo, and Ana then proceeded to sever contacts with other family members and seemingly, disappeared from sight. The parents called Silvia and Carlos on occasion, but never again did they come to visit the children in their foster homes. The parents had moved from where they had been living and CPS never knew where they had gone. CPS asked Silvia and Carlos to ask their parents to contact CPS, but the parents never did. CPS issued a warrant for Ana's arrest, but she never was located.

What Had Gone Wrong?

Of the three children, Ana was the most upset at being separated from her parents. Change was particularly difficult for her. She clearly was unhappy in the group home. When the psychologist had interviewed her, she had downplayed the problems that had existed with her parents and their alcoholism.

There was nothing in the psychologist's report to indicate the parents would try to kidnap their children. It seems that the parents also tried to lure Silvia and Carlos away from their foster homes as well, but were unsuccessful.

It is clear that the psychologist's recommendation that the children be placed in foster homes where they would receive individual attention was not followed, especially in Ana's case. There were five other girls in Ana's group home and they teased her incessantly because of her low functioning and general lack of interest in relating to others. The house parent, Martha Ortiz, also complained about all the things that Ana was unable to do by herself.

Separating the siblings, as the psychologist recommended, does not seem to have been a good idea. Ana could have used the support from her siblings. As it turns out, the separation was hard on Silvia and Carlos as well. However, finding a foster home that could have taken in all three siblings, no doubt, would have been difficult for CPS (see Exhibit 6.3).

Mental Health Services for Silvia

Within six months of the adjudication/disposition hearing, Nancy, Advocacy Services' senior attorney, was appointed to represent Silvia and Carlos. A major purpose of the representation was to ensure that the children received appropriate educational and psychological services to meet their needs.

It was at this point that I entered the case in order to try to address Silvia and Carlos' educational needs. After reviewing Silvia's school records and talking with her, I called the school that Silvia was

---

EXHIBIT 6.3.
Research on Separating Siblings

Twenty-five percent of the separated sibling groups had four or more placements, but none of the intact sibling groups had this many placements. Overall, the healthiest children were most likely to be placed together while children who most needed the support of siblings were least likely to receive it. (Aldridge & Cautley, 1976)

attending to request a special education evaluation for her, which, fortunately, the psychologist readily agreed to initiate. I had planned on attending the IEP meeting when the evaluation was completed, but on the day the meeting was scheduled, there were torrential rains and many of the freeways and streets were flooded. With the rain, the flooding, and, consequently, the horrendous traffic problems that ensued, it would have been hard enough to get to the meeting, given the distance from my home and office, and I was not sure whether, after the meeting, I would be able to get home successfully that night.

Rather than attend the IEP meeting for Silvia, I contacted the school psychologist with whom I previously had spoken and told him of my situation. I discussed with him his assessment findings and the recommendations he thought would be made for Silvia at the meeting. He indicated that he was fairly certain Silvia would be found eligible for special education services as a student with a learning disability in the area of reading. At sixteen years old, she was reading at the first grade level. Her math scores were better, at the mid-fifth grade level. The psychologist's evaluation took into account her bilingual background, chaotic home life, and numerous absences from school over the years, but still concluded, "[t]here is sufficient evidence however to indicate that she has a specific learning disability which affects her functioning in both languages and is not the result of her experiential background."

I told the psychologist that I supported this recommendation, but I also had concerns about Silvia's mental health. I let him know that the court-ordered psychological evaluation found Silvia in need of psychological counseling and that her mental health problems no doubt were impacting her functioning at school. He told me Silvia was not a behavior problem at school, which was no surprise to me, since, from my conversation with her as well as Nancy's description of their interactions I knew she was a lovely, well-behaved young woman. I discussed with him that the psychologist who provided a court-ordered evaluation of the family found her to be in emotional distress, that she worried constantly, was often afraid, and cried easily. Since I could not attend the meeting, I requested that he discuss Silvia's emotional needs with the IEP team and request that a referral to the local department of mental health (DMH) be made for her. The psychologist told me he would discuss my concerns with the IEP team and raise the possibility of making a DMH referral.

Intervention

I called the psychologist back after the IEP meeting to find out what had occurred. He relayed that the IEP team had indeed found Silvia eligible for special education and that she would begin receiving special education services for part of her school day to address her learning disability, which affected her reading, spelling, and writing. When I inquired about the referral to DMH, the psychologist told me he wanted to see the court-ordered evaluation first describing her mental health problems, and that he would be providing counseling services for her at this point, which the IEP team had authorized.

Nancy and I reviewed the family's court-ordered evaluation and selected portions that we felt would be helpful to the psychologist in understanding Silvia's mental health needs, but would not breach the confidentiality of the other family members. I then sent this information to him.

I called the psychologist about a week later. He said he had reviewed the material I sent him and now he would send the referral to DMH. After this conversation, I called the program head at DMH and let him know that a referral would be coming and gave him some information about Silvia's needs.

About two months later, about the time I thought DMH would have completed its mental health evaluation of Silvia and would be scheduling an IEP meeting to discuss the findings and what services, hopefully, they would be recommending for her, I called the school psychologist back. He told me that he never had made the referral to DMH, and, instead, still was giving Silvia weekly counseling. He now agreed that, based on his work with Silvia, her mental health needs warranted a referral to DMH.

There were a couple of other concerns the psychologist wanted to discuss related to the referral. First, he told me that Luisa Gonzalez, Silvia's foster mother, did not believe she had the authority to sign the DMH referral form, a form that was needed for this referral to be accepted by DMH. Second, he said Luisa Gonzalez expressed concern at the possibility of having to transport Silvia to a county clinic to receive the mental health services. I told him the foster mother did have the authority to sign the referral form and the school district simply had to appoint her as the surrogate parent for Silvia, since her birth parents could not be located (IDEA, 2004). Furthermore, special education law (Interagency Responsibilities, 2004) required that the school district either provide transportation for a special education student to receive IEP-authorized mental health services, or to reimburse the foster parent for her transportation costs (see Exhibit 6.4).

A week later, a student law clerk at Advocacy Services called the psychologist again to see whether the DMH referral had been made and learned that the psychologist still had not made the referral. Pam Marx, staff attorney at Advocacy Services, started working on the case and called the psychologists' supervisor to discuss the importance of a DMH referral for Silvia. In my next phone conversation with the psychologist, he told me he would send the DMH referral form to the foster parent's home. Pam then visited Silvia in her foster home and, since Silvia had just turned eighteen, told her that as an adult she could legally sign the referral form instead of her foster parent, which she did and returned it to the school psychologist the next day. Pam then followed up a few days later by calling the school psychologist who then told her that he had indeed processed the DMH referral.

About two months later, when the DMH evaluation should have been completed, Pam called the psychologist back to discuss the scheduling of an IEP meeting. At that time, Pam learned that the school psychologist had retired and, in fact, had never sent the referral to DMH. Pam shared this information with Nancy and me. We were furious at having been misled and, furthermore, that the psychologist's failure to make the referral resulted in further delay in obtaining mental health services for Silvia. Pam then spoke with the psychologist who had taken over the caseload of the former psychologist and she

---

EXHIBIT 6.4.
Rights of Surrogate Parents

Appointed surrogate parents have the same rights as a child's parent to consent to special education assessments and implementation of services. (IDEA, 2004)

agreed to process the DMH referral, which, thankfully, she immediately did.

Intervention

At the IEP meeting, which I attended hoping finally to get mental health services in place for Silvia, the DMH evaluator recommended mental health services for her because she was quite depressed and had considerable anxiety. The report stated, "Silvia constantly worries about her family's welfare. She admits to not being able to stop worrying; not having any enjoyment in life and feeling depressed or sad in general, her feelings are reserved and her affect is subdued."

The recommended mental health services were individual and/or group psychological therapy at least once a week. A psychiatric evaluation also was recommended to determine if she required medication to relieve her symptoms, and, if so, medication monitoring would be provided. Family therapy was offered as well, presumably with the foster family. These services then were written on her IEP along with reimbursement of transportation costs to her foster mother who would provide the transportation to and from the mental health clinic. Silvia then started receiving individual psychological therapy from a department of mental health clinic, and her therapy sessions seemed to be quite helpful in relieving some of her depression and anxiety.

What Had Gone Wrong?

A referral and mental health evaluation that, by state law (Interagency Responsibilities for Related Services, 2004), should have taken no more than seventy-five days ended up taking eight months. Why had the psychologist not followed through with the referral for the mental health evaluation? Initially, he decided to provide her with school counseling, presumably to determine the extent of her psychological problems. As a first step, this was appropriate, particularly before he had documentation of the extent of Silvia's mental health needs. The state law, in fact, requires that in particular. It specifies, prior to making a referral to DMH for a student with an IEP, a local education agency (i.e., Silvia's school district) first must have provided school counseling and determined that the counseling was not adequate to meet the child's needs (Interagency Responsibilities for

Related Services, 2004). However, a school district does have the option of making a DMH referral without having provided school counseling if the district knew or had documentation that the child's mental health problems were of a sufficient magnitude that school counseling would not be adequate. Once the psychologist had both first hand knowledge and documentation of Silvia's extensive mental health needs, the DMH referral should have been made promptly, which it was not.

It really never became clear whether the psychologist's lack of follow through was an indication of his resistance to making the referral in the first place, his lack of know-how in doing so, or whether he had really started his retirement before the official date and just stopped doing his job. The sad part is that Silvia was not getting professional help with her depression during this time. While the failure of this particular school psychologist may have been a unique situation, there are just too many ways that those who have important responsibilities to vulnerable children contribute to widening the cracks in an already compromised system.

Advocacy Considerations

One of the issues that Silvia's foster parent raised was her legal right to sign the referral form so that the school district could refer Silvia's case and records to DMH. Did the foster mother have the authority to sign the referral to DMH for Silvia? Under special education law, a child's parent has the authority to sign consent for assessments and for services. In Silvia's case, the whereabouts of her parent were not known. The U.S. Congress contemplated this type of situation when it originally passed the IDEA; what was required was for a school district to appoint a surrogate parent to sign the needed consents for such a child (IDEA, 2004). Silvia's foster parent would have been the obvious surrogate parent to appoint. The child's social worker, as an employee of the county (and agent of the state) was not eligible for this role (IDEA, 2004).

Once Silvia became eighteen, under state law (Special Education Programs, 2005), she had the right to sign her own consents for referral, assessment, and services as an adult. She then no longer needed a surrogate parent to be appointed (see Exhibit 6.5).

EXHIBIT 6.5.
When a Special Education Student Becomes an Adult

Once a special education student reaches the age of majority, the student may sign his or her consent for assessment and IEP unless. . . . (Special Education Programs, 2005)

Special Education Services for Carlos

Carlos, at nine years old, could not read in either English or Spanish. After talking over what course of action we should take to enhance his development in this crucial area at our weekly staff meeting, I contacted the psychologist at Carlos' school to request that Carlos be evaluated for special education services. The school psychologist seemed resistant to evaluating Carlos, even though he already had done some preliminary screening of his reading skills, based on a referral from Carlos' teacher. Not surprisingly, the psychologist had found Carlos' reading skills to be quite low. The reason the psychologist gave to justify his hesitation to initiate a full evaluation was that Carlos had missed a significant number of days of school over the years and, the psychologist speculated, perhaps his low achievement in reading was attributable to that rather than to a learning disability. The psychologist's concern was reasonable. However, Carlos now had been in this school for about seven months with perfect attendance and was not making much progress at all in reading. He was in the fourth grade; based on his age, he should have been in the fifth, but previously had been retained.

Intervention

This current school district was sending Carlos to a first and second grade combination class for ninety minutes each day to try to improve his ability to read and write. This approach did not seem to be improving his skills in reading. I had concerns about how Carlos' already low self-esteem would fare, with him being sent to a classroom with children who were much younger than he was for part of his school day.

Requesting an Evaluation for Special Education for Carlos

The psychologist continued to be resistant to initiating an evaluation for Carlos, so I told him I would put my request in writing and that if the school district refused to act on it, our office would file for a special education hearing on Carlos' behalf in order to have the district assess him. Following my conversation with the psychologist, I sent a formal request to the school district requesting that Carlos be evaluated (see Exhibit 6.6).

Obviously, the psychologist had a change of mind because he completed the testing promptly and the district's coordinator of special education set up Carlos' IEP meeting. The question at the IEP meeting was whether Carlos was eligible for special education services on the basis of a specific learning disability. Based on the psychologist's testing, Carlos clearly met the eligibility requirements for a learning disability (Special Education Programs, 2005). But the psychologist also reported that in the six years that Carlos had gone to school, in terms of the number of days he actually attended, he only had been in school a total of three years. Was Carlos' inability to read related to a learning disability or to lack of instruction? Even though the psychologist was hesitant to make Carlos eligible for special education services, the IEP team as a whole, including the Coordinator of Special Education, felt that the assessment data clearly was strong enough to indicate that Carlos indeed had a learning disability (see Exhibit 6.7).

EXHIBIT 6.6.
Let the School District Know You Will File for a Hearing

If the school refuses to initiate an assessment for special education for a child whose skills do not improve with instruction, let the district know that you will file for a special education hearing in order to have the child evaluated. If the district then does not provide an assessment plan and consent for assessment, follow through and file for a hearing. Seek advice and/or representation from an agency that provides free or low-cost legal services in the area of special education law.

EXHIBIT 6.7.
Specific Learning Disability

Specific learning disability "means a disorder in one or more of the basic psychological processes involved in understanding or in using language, spoken or written, that may manifest itself in an imperfect ability to listen, think, speak, read, write, spell, or to do mathematical calculations. . . . Such term includes such conditions as perceptual disabilities, brain injury, minimal brain dysfunction, dyslexia, and developmental aphasia. . . . Such term does not include learning problems that are primarily the result of visual, hearing, or motor disabilities, of mental retardation, of emotional disturbance or of environmental, cultural, or economic disadvantage." (IDEA, 2004, §1402(30))

Advocacy Considerations

Carlos required intensive instruction and practice in reading. This presented a dilemma because the school district was not set up to provide the intensive instruction Carlos needed as part of the regular fourth grade program. The only options presented were having Carlos attend the first/second grade combination class for ninety minutes a day or make him eligible for special education services. Since he had not been progressing in the first/second grade class and there were serious concerns about his self-esteem in that setting, we decided to try the special education option. Currently, there are additional intensive general education interventions available in some school districts for children who fail to respond to instruction in academic areas based on the most recent reauthorization of the federal special education law (IDEA, 2004).

Carlos Receives Special Education Services

Intervention

The IEP meeting was held in the summer. Carlos started receiving instruction in the special education classroom in the fall.

I went to observe the class to make sure it was well run and that we had made the correct decision for Carlos. There were fourteen students in the class. I watched Carlos and a group of six other students work with the classroom aide on a reading, spelling, and word meaning activity. The classroom aide showed a student in the group a flashcard with a word written on it. The student then had to read the word and say what it meant. The word on the flashcard Carlos was shown was "hero." He had trouble with the word, so the aide gave him some help trying to sound it out. Other students ultimately helped Carlos read the word and come up with the definition. The students also worked on spelling and writing the words.

I felt the activity the aide was working on was too advanced for Carlos at his very low reading level. I also had some concern with the high activity level of the students working with the aide. She constantly had to discipline and refocus them. Carlos seemed quite distracted by the other students and the aide did not seem to notice Carlos' lack of involvement in the activity.

I briefly talked to the teacher who said she would start sending Carlos to the regular fourth grade class in a couple of weeks for math, physical education, art, and music. She said Carlos was working in a first grade book for reading. She told me that she had known Carlos because, prior to his IEP meeting, he used to stop by her classroom.

I spent some time talking with Carlos. He told me he was fine being in the special education class, but that most of his friends, with whom he played at nutrition and lunch, were in the regular fourth grade class. I decided I would come back to observe Carlos again in a couple weeks and then decide if we needed to make an adjustment in his program. I was thinking it might be better (academically and socially) if Carlos were placed in the regular fourth grade classroom with some intensive individualized instruction and support in reading (see Exhibit 6.8).

EXHIBIT 6.8.
Classroom Observation

If you cannot observe a prospective school placement for a student with a disability prior to the student being placed in that school setting, it is important to observe the classroom once the placement is made to determine whether, in fact, it is appropriate for the child.

Unfortunately for this plan, Carlos was moved from the foster home he was in and placed in the home of his aunt and uncle a short time after. Consequently, I never was able to return and do more observation of his program at this school.

Advocacy Considerations

The district offered a full-day special education class for Carlos. It was a class for students who had learning disabilities, although, as it turned out, there were students in that class with attention and mild to moderate behavior problems as well, which was not unusual for this type of special education program. Had I had the opportunity to return to the class and if I again felt that the behavior of certain students made it hard for Carlos to learn in that setting, I would have called for another IEP meeting to discuss other options for Carlos. One of the options I likely would have requested would have been a placement in a regular fourth grade class with one-to-one instruction for Carlos with a reading specialist.

Sibling Visits and a Social Security Card

Within two months from the time that Nancy was appointed to represent Silvia and Carlos, the social worker who originally had been assigned to their case was transferred. A new social worker should have been assigned immediately. Pam, the Advocacy Services staff attorney, called the CPS office trying to find out who the new social worker was and, to her dismay, learned that no one, in fact, had yet been assigned. Having no social worker on their case caused serious problems for Silvia and Carlos. They wanted to visit each other, but were prevented from doing so by their respective foster parents (in accordance with CPS policy) without authorization from their social worker. In addition, Silvia wanted to get a job, but needed a social security card to do so. Since she was not born in the United States, a CPS social worker was needed to facilitate obtaining a social security card for her.

What Had Gone Wrong?

Pam called the CPS office periodically to check on whether a social worker had been assigned yet, but learned that the clerk for this

CPS office, whose job it was to assign social workers to cases, had been out on leave for several months and no one was taking over her responsibilities. Unfortunately, Silvia and Carlos were unable to visit with each other during this period of time and Silvia was unable to get a job. In this instance, the cracks the siblings were falling through were forged by bureaucratic dysfunction.

Using a Court Order to Request Sibling Visits

There was a court review hearing during this period of time that Pam attended as the attorney from our office. It was the job of the social worker on the case to submit a report to the court. However, since there was no social worker, no court report was submitted. The juvenile court judge was quite upset at the fact that neither was there a social worker on the case nor a court report submitted about how the children were faring. Pam requested from this judge a court order to allow sibling visits, which the judge quickly granted. However, without the report or a social worker assigned to Silvia and Carlos, the judge deferred the hearing to two months later with an order for CPS to assign a social worker who would visit the children and submit a report by the next hearing.

Within two weeks of the court hearing, Pam learned that two social workers were now sharing the case and would be visiting Silvia and Carlos prior to the next court hearing. Sibling visits also were to be arranged. However, when Pam called one of the social workers a couple of weeks later, she learned that Silvia and Carlos had not yet visited each other. The problem, according to the social worker, was related to CPS forms that each foster parent had to complete before the sibling visits could take place. Although the social worker claimed to have sent out these forms, neither foster parent had received them. Pam made it clear that there was a standing court order allowing sibling visits and the social worker was responsible for arranging the visits. If there were forms to be signed, then it was the social worker's responsibility to make sure that this was done promptly. Finally, seven months after Advocacy Services had been assigned to work on the case, the children were able to visit with each other and spend the night at one of their foster homes.

Obtaining a social security card for Silvia took several more months of advocacy by Pam, before Silvia finally got a social security card.

What Had Gone Wrong?

There clearly was a management problem at the CPS office. This problem was further exacerbated by the fact that CPS, like many CPS agencies around the county, had a perpetual shortage of social workers and office staff (Child Welfare League of America, 2002; Gunderson & Osborne, 2001). In this case, the person responsible for assigning social workers to cases was out for several months and her job responsibilities were not properly delegated to anyone else. CPS not only failed to arrange for sibling visits but also had failed to visit the children on a monthly basis as the law required.

Carlos Moves in with Relatives

Silvia and Carlos' aunt and uncle decided that they wanted Carlos to live with them. So without any warning or preparation for the aunt and uncle regarding the difficulties that Carlos' living with them might present, Carlos was moved from the foster home, in which he had been for nine months, into their home. At a court hearing, Pam, who was solely English speaking, met Carlos' aunt, Juanita Fernandez, who was solely Spanish speaking. Juanita was accompanied by her twenty-year-old daughter, Susana, who was bilingual, and learned that Carlos was enrolled in the local school in their community, but was not receiving any special education services.

Shortly after the court hearing, I called Susana to discuss why Carlos currently was not receiving any special education services. She told me that her mother wanted Carlos to be placed in the same school, and on the same track, as her own children and that she was told that the only way Carlos could receive special education services was to be placed in a different school. The reason for this, the aunt had been told, was that all the special education classes at the school that Carlos' cousins attended were full. Although Carlos now was placed at the same school as his cousins, in a regular fifth grade class, he was not placed in the same track, because there was no space. Therefore, Carlos' school year and semester breaks did not correspond with his cousins.

Securing Special Education Services for Carlos

I called 57th St. Elementary School, the school that Carlos and his cousins were attending, and spoke with the coordinator of bilingual services, since she was the person with whom the aunt had interacted while enrolling Carlos. I asked her about the possibility of changing Carlos' track to conform to his cousin's as well as providing special education services for him. After talking with her, I called the school psychologist who provided services to this school, twice a week, and explained to her Carlos' academic and mental health needs. I reminded her that an IEP meeting should take place within thirty days from the time Carlos enrolled in the school (Special Education Programs, 2005). She said she would set up the IEP meeting but wanted to see the evaluation of Carlos from the previous school district, which I agreed to send her.

To my surprise, the coordinator of bilingual services called me back the same day. She told me that the resource specialist would evaluate Carlos the following day and, subsequently, they would place him in the Resource Special Program (RSP) at the school, a less than half-day special education class. The remainder of his day would be in the regular fifth-grade class. They also would allow Carlos to attend the Resource Program during his intersession (when his regular session was off track).

I called Carlos' cousin Susana and brought her up-to-date on what the coordinator had conveyed. A concern she shared with me was that her mother felt Carlos was not always being honest about the homework he had. Her mother wanted the teacher to inform her about Carlos' homework so she did not have to rely solely on what Carlos told her.

The next day the resource specialist evaluated Carlos. Following the evaluation, I received a call from the coordinator of bilingual services. The coordinator informed me that a space had just opened up in the full day special education class at their school for students of Carlos' age. She was very positive about the special education teacher who taught this class.

Advocacy Considerations

Getting Carlos placed in an appropriate special education class and on the same track as his cousins' primarily required continued contact with appropriate school personnel and knowledge of his rights. It also seemed that once the school district realized the severity of Carlos' reading disability and that an advocate from a law office was working on his behalf, only then a place in the special day class opened up.

Special Education Placement

Intervention

Shortly after Carlos was placed in the special day class, I went to observe the class to see how he was doing. There were thirteen students in this class with a teacher and a part-time aide, who left at 12:30 p.m. everyday. The students were doing an art project of making Christmas decorations, since it was the week before the winter break. Carlos was actively engaged in the art project, as were the other students, and he was wearing his glasses, which he had been hesitant to do in the past.

The class seemed well organized and student work, classroom activities, and the class schedule were proudly displayed on the bulletin boards. I spent a little time talking to the teacher who indicated that Carlos was doing well in the class and was accepted by the other students. She told me that his reading and spelling skills were at the first-grade level and his math skills were much higher. Math was Carlos' favorite subject, she reported, and he was working on division problems in her class. Her major concern was that Carlos lacked confidence in his ability to do his schoolwork. He wanted someone to sit with him and help him do his work, although it was work she knew he could do by himself.

I talked with Carlos' cousin after my observation at the school. She reported that things were going well at home and that her aunt was considering becoming a legal guardian for Carlos. This was good news; he seemed to be well placed in his school program and perhaps he might have some stability in his home life as well.

Placement with Relatives Ends

About a month and a half after my classroom observation, Pam was talking to Carlos and Silvia's social worker when she dashed our hopes of stability for Carlos with his aunt and uncle. She told Pam that Juanita, his aunt, had reported to the social worker that Carlos was refusing to do his homework or to follow her directions. His aunt said that Carlos had told her that he wanted to be with his parents and Juanita was afraid they would come and take him away. Worst of all, she said, Carlos told her he wanted to kill someone and so she felt she no longer could provide a home for him. Consequently, Juanita asked the social worker to find a foster home for Carlos as soon as possible. The social worker told the aunt she would refer Carlos for psychological counseling and hoped this would encourage her to keep Carlos longer, but the social worker did not think that Juanita would change her mind.

Pam had another conversation with the social worker, who informed her that Juanita had requested that Carlos be placed in a foster home far away from her home so his parents would not know where he was. She relayed that Carlos and Silvia's father had been calling Carlos and telling him that he was going to join the army. This information presumably worried Carlos. His oldest sister, Ana, who had run away from her group home and now was living with their parents, also called Carlos and encouraged him to run away. The aunt was worried the parents would come and take Carlos.

What Had Gone Wrong?

It seems foolhardy to have placed Carlos with his aunt and uncle without any preparation for them about the kinds of problems they would be confronting with this living arrangement. The aunt and uncle seemed to believe that Carlos should have been grateful that they took him in and, therefore, not cause them any problems. In addition, it did not make sense that Carlos did not have any psychological counseling to help him with the difficult transition to his aunt and uncle's home as well as family therapy to help them all live together better. The ongoing intrusion of Silvia and Carlos' parents in their lives obviously was difficult for all of them and they needed help in dealing with it.

IEP Meeting

I called Carlos' teacher about scheduling an IEP meeting for Carlos since it was well overdue. I also hoped that Carlos' aunt would change her mind, but his teacher was not encouraged. Although it appeared that Carlos would be moving soon, I still felt it was important that we had an IEP meeting for him. I wanted to request a referral for mental health services from DMH through the IEP process. I thought these mental health services particularly would be important for Carlos given the imminent change in his living place and school. My feelings were reinforced when the teacher informed me that Carlos was no longer doing his homework and when he was in school, he constantly was asking to go to the bathroom. The teacher said that both of these were new behaviors she had not seen before.

The IEP meeting was held in Carlos' classroom and was attended by Juanita. I had an opportunity to talk with Carlos before the meeting. He told me, in a somewhat disjointed way, that he was having trouble sleeping at night and frequently got up and walked around because he was worried. I asked him if he would like someone to talk to who could help him with his problems and he said he would.

At the IEP meeting, the teacher reported on Carlos' performance in class, which seemed to be fine until he came back from winter break. I requested a referral for mental health services from DMH. Everyone at the meeting agreed that Carlos would benefit from mental health services and that his emotional problems were negatively affecting his ability to function in school and at home. The only question that was raised was on the timing of the referral since Carlos would be changing school districts shortly. I told the other members of the IEP team that since Carlos would still be in the same county, it would be a good idea to make the referral now and start the mental health assessment timeline ticking. The IEP team members agreed this was a good plan and delineated it on the IEP. I hoped DMH would not require a new referral once Carlos changed school districts. Within two weeks after the IEP meeting, Carlos was moved to a foster home.

Starting a New School

Carlos moved into his new foster home. He started attending the local school in his new neighborhood when he was one month shy of his tenth birthday.

Intervention

He was enrolled in a full-day special education class for students with learning disabilities. Interestingly, the district accelerated Carlos to the sixth grade in accordance with his age.

The Struggle to Obtain Mental Health Services for Carlos

I called the program head at DMH to apprise him that Carlos was no longer residing in the same school district. To my dismay, the program head told me that he never had received the DMH referral from the school district that Carlos had attended while living with his aunt and uncle. I decided to try and figure out where the referral was and why it never was sent to DMH. I called one of the head psychologists for the school district and learned that the psychologist who had attended Carlos' IEP meeting should have made the referral, but, as it turns out, had never made one before and, unfortunately, did not follow through on it. A month and a half later, the referral landed on the head psychologist's desk and, by that time, Carlos was no longer in the district. Since several months had passed since Carlos had left this school district, the head psychologist said it would be more appropriate for Carlos' new school district to make the referral to DMH. In fact, he had already sent the new school district the information on Carlos that needed to be forwarded to DMH.

My call to the psychologist at Carlos' new school district also was not encouraging. She wanted me to provide her with a written justification that Carlos needed these DMH services. I realized that this psychologist had never previously made a referral to DMH either, so I told her what the procedures were and that our office would provide her with the information she wanted. Pam put together a letter describing Carlos' history and his current mental health problems and sent it to her. About ten days later, Pam called the psychologist and was gratified to learn that she had actually sent a referral packet to DMH for Carlos.

What Had Gone Wrong?

The state law that provided mental health services to special education students had been in existence for many years when we were trying to obtain those services for Carlos through this process. Obviously, there was a need for training of school psychologists in how to refer students for these services.

Advocacy Considerations

Constant monitoring at every step of the referral process was necessary to ensure referrals for the mental health services would in fact be made. In retrospect, I realize that I should have been even more vigilant in my monitoring of the referrals.

Silvia Moves with Her Foster Parent to an Adjoining County

At the end of the school semester, Silvia's foster family moved into a new home in an adjoining county. Arrangements had been made ahead of time with CPS for Silvia to move with the Gonzalez family. However, Silvia and Carlos' social worker had to inspect the new house before Silvia was able to move with the family. This took a bit of time but the social worker eventually inspected the home and gave her okay for Silvia to live there.

IEP Meeting in New School District

Silvia started attending school in the new school district. An IEP meeting was promptly held the following month to review her educational needs. It was attended by Pam from our office.. The primary purpose of this meeting was to determine if the part-time special education program Silvia had been in at her previous school was still an appropriate type of setting for her. The other issue was to ensure that Silvia would continue to receive mental health services in this new county.

Getting Silvia's mental health services up and going, however, took some effort. At the meeting, Pam conveyed that Silvia had been receiving mental health services in the previous county and that these services were written on her IEP. The new school district indicated that there was a six-month waiting list in this county for these mental health services.

Advocacy Efforts to Restore Mental Health Services

After the meeting, Pam wrote a letter to the head of the DMH program in the new county delineating Silvia's need for these services and that putting her on a waiting list for the services was a violation of the law. This letter attained the desired results.

Intervention

DMH immediately initiated Silvia's mental health services. Silvia's foster mother drove Silvia to the clinic so she could begin receiving these services.

Several months later, rather abruptly, Silvia stopped receiving the mental health services. It was not quite clear what the problem actually was. There seemed to have been some confusion between Silvia, the school district, and DMH regarding these services. Nevertheless, Pam contacted DMH and the services quickly were resumed.

Advocacy Considerations

Pam's strategy was effective—writing a letter to the head of the DMH program and clearly specifying that putting Silvia on a waiting list was a violation of the law. Pam's vigilance on this case and Silvia's notifying Pam when services stopped helped to restore mental health services very quickly.

Carlos' Behavior Deteriorates

During this time, Carlos' behavior at the foster home had deteriorated to such an extent that his foster mother decided she no longer wanted to care for him. He did not know it yet, but she wanted him removed from her home at the end of the school year, which was just a couple of weeks away. She felt that Carlos was just too aggressive. He frequently tried to hit or choke the other children in the home, threw a skateboard at them, and had torn out her outdoor plants.

What Had Gone Wrong?

One of the problems that, no doubt, contributed to Carlos' poor behavior was that he was not having regular visits with his sister. Once Carlos was in the new foster home, the foster mother, at first, did not want his sister to have the address because she was fearful that Carlos' parents would find him and kidnap him. Furthermore, Silvia was not calling him very often because the telephone bill at her foster home had been very high from her previous calls and, consequently, she felt uncomfortable making any calls. Toward the end of his stay at this foster home, the visitation and phone call schedule was worked out, but it was too late (see Exhibit 6.9).

Placing Silvia and Carlos in the Same Foster Home

The school semester ended and so did Carlos' placement in the foster home and the school district he had been attending. At that time, with Silvia's urging, her foster mother agreed, on a trial basis, to care for Carlos in her home. Carlos was now one month past his eleventh birthday. Silvia, at this time, had been living with the Gonzalez foster family for over two years and had become very attached to Luisa, her foster mother.

Intervention

Once Carlos was placed in the same foster home as his sister, his behavior improved. He seemed genuinely happy for the first time in a very long time.

Initiating Services for Carlos

Carlos' placement in his sister's foster home occurred in the beginning of summer. Pam encouraged Luisa Gonzalez to sign Carlos up for summer school, and facilitated the enrollment by contacting the school and working out all the arrangements.

Pam also tried to establish mental health services for Carlos. A phone call to the DMH representative did not much advance things.

EXHIBIT 6.9.
The Effect of Separating Siblings on Permanency

. . . [S]eparating sibling groups may contribute to further disruption in the form of multiple placements and ultimately failure to achieve permanency, as children use one of the few tools they have—negative behaviors—to attempt to disrupt placements and be reunited with brothers and sisters. (Casey Family Programs, 2003)

The representative said that the school district psychologist had to make a new referral. Luckily, however, since a mental health referral had been specified on Carlos' IEP when he was still living with his aunt and uncle, and there had not been a new IEP since then, the new school district agreed immediately to make the referral to DMH.

Intervention

Shortly after the referral was made, mental health services finally started for Carlos. It had taken much too long for these services to begin, from the time I first requested them when Carlos was living with his aunt and uncle. Nevertheless, we were happy that Carlos now would be receiving mental health services.

IEP Meeting in New School District

In the fall, Pam attended the entry IEP meeting for Carlos in this school district. Carlos had just started the seventh grade and the reports at this meeting indicated he was functioning at the first and second grade level in all subjects, except for math, which was at the third to fourth grade level (lower than previously reported).

Intervention

Pam requested specific tutoring services to help improve Carlos' reading skills, which the district agreed to provide him after school twice a week. We hoped the tutoring services would give Carlos the additional support he needed to improve his ability to read. In addition, Pam requested that Carlos receive an evaluation from the district's speech and language specialist to identify whether a speech and language deficit in Spanish contributed to Carlos' difficulty in learning to read and express himself well in English.

IEP Meeting for Silvia

At an IEP meeting for Silvia, Pam expressed considerable concern about Silvia's continuing failure to improve in her reading skills. Silvia was moving toward the time when she would be on her own, and expected to support herself. Yet, her word identification and word attack skills were still around the first grade level, even though her passage comprehension skills were somewhat higher, at the mid-third-grade level.

Intervention

Because of Pam's insistence on this issue, the school district agreed to provide a peer tutor for Silvia to work on a special adult literacy program twice a week.

Advocacy Considerations

Nothing more would have been done to improve Silvia's skills in reading had Pam not pressed the issue.

CPS Wants to Terminate Jurisdiction

Pam learned that CPS intended to transfer Silvia and Carlos' juvenile court case to the county in which both children now were living and, in addition, to recommend that the juvenile court terminate jurisdiction for Silvia at the end of the school year. When Pam shared this information with Nancy and me, we were not pleased with either of these recommendations. Pam expressed our concerns in a letter she sent to the social worker. She argued in the letter that maintaining the case in the original county provided important continuity for the children, particularly in terms of Advocacy Services continuing to represent them. Furthermore, their aunt and uncle lived in this county and they were the only family members with whom the children had any contact.

Regarding completely terminating jurisdiction for Silvia, Pam argued that even though Silvia might have the credits to graduate from high school in seven months, she was not prepared at all to start supporting herself. Furthermore, she had missed so much schooling over the years that she dearly needed to remain in high school for as much time as was possible. Silvia clearly was willing to remain in school an extra year and her IEP team thought it was a good idea.

Pam's letter proved effective. CPS did not try to transfer jurisdiction of their case to the county in which the siblings were now living nor push for termination of Silvia's case, thus allowing her to remain in high school an extra year.

Advocacy Considerations

Under special education law, a student with disabilities may remain in high school until his or her twenty-second birthday if the student does not graduate. Pam made sure, through the IEP process, that Silvia was not graduated prematurely. As it turned out, Silvia did not graduate high school until she was twenty. Furthermore, Pam's letter to Silvia and Carlos' social worker was effective in preventing CPS from trying to transfer the jurisdiction on their case to another county and to enable Silvia to remain a dependent until she graduated from high school. Since federal child welfare funding is not available for a foster youth past his or her eighteenth birthday, the county had to pick up all of the cost to keep her in her foster home until she was twenty.

CONCLUSION

Silvia had the good fortune to spend her entire time in foster care with one foster family. However, Carlos was not so fortunate. He was in two different foster homes, lived for a short period with his aunt and uncle, and finally, because of Silvia's good relationship with her foster family, was placed in the foster home with his sister. In Carlos' case, he clearly needed the security and constant presence of his sister in his life.

In retrospect, the decision to place Carlos with his aunt and uncle and cousins, while well intentioned, was a recipe for failure. There was no immediate support for the family when Carlos' emotional and behavioral problems became known. Neither was there any guidance and support when the possibility of Silvia and Carlos' parents luring Carlos away arose. Relative, or kinship, foster placements must include appropriate support services, when needed, to make such placements viable.

Finally, representation of a child frequently requires ensuring that the child receives appropriate educational and mental health services. Availability of these services frequently differs in different locales. When home placements change, the ability to ensure continuity of educational and mental health services may be difficult, as was the case for Silvia and Carlos, as well as the other children described in this book.

SUMMARY

The purpose of this chapter was to show how the failure to place siblings together could be a recipe for disaster. This was the situation when Carlos was not placed in the same foster home as his sister, Silvia, the person who had provided stability for him in his life. This chapter also demonstrates that placing a youngster with his relatives is not always the right decision, particularly when the relatives are not given supportive services to help them understand the emotional trauma that the child placed in their home is experiencing. In addition, the chapter describes the difficulty of accessing appropriate services for children at the upper elementary and high school levels whose reading skills still are at a first grade level. Furthermore, the chapter makes clear that accessing mental health services for youth in foster care continues to be a serious problem and the problem compounds as children move from one home placement to another and into other counties.

Chapter 7

Robert:
Living at the County
Emergency Shelter

INTRODUCTION

Foster youths have been found to have higher rates of depression, poorer social skills, lower adaptive functioning, and more externalizing behavioral problems, such as aggression and impulsivity, than do other children (Clausen, Landsverk, Ganger, Chadwick, & Litrownik, 1998; U.S. Department of Health and Human Services [DHHS], 2003). When these behaviors, such as unprovoked aggressive outbursts coupled with inappropriate sexual behavior, are extreme, it may be very difficult to maintain foster youths in standard foster care settings, such as traditional foster homes, group homes, and residential treatment facilities. Finding a permanent placement for these youths may require alternative and creative solutions.

Robert's case focuses on the problem of not providing a child's parent with the necessary, ongoing, and sufficiently intensive services that might allow the child to remain in the home. This led to Robert's placement in living situations that were unable to adequately address his tremendous needs for care, mental health treatment, and education. This chapter considers the grave difficulties of caring for a youngster whose disabilities and the kinds of services he required were not well understood, particularly as he became an adolescent and moved toward the time when he would "age out" of the foster care system.

The Systematic Mistreatment of Children in the Foster Care System
© 2007 by The Haworth Press, Taylor & Francis Group. All rights reserved.
doi:10.1300/5136_07   *147*

Robert, an African-American male, could not be stabilized in his out-of-home foster care placements. He went in and out of one group home or residential treatment facility after another. There were several attempts to place him with his mother. His aggressive behavior seemed to increase significantly with each placement change. As he became older and larger and actively sought out sexual experiences, his placement options diminished significantly.

The county where Robert lived did not have such options as wraparound or therapeutic foster homes. These are placement options intended to provide intensive services in a least restrictive environment to youth with severe emotional or behavioral disorders. Wraparound is a community-based, team-driven process that involves the child and family and provides individualized services and supports to meet the unique needs of children and families (Burchard, Burns, & Burchard, 2002). Foster youths with severe emotional and behavioral problems and their families are provided the array of services and supports that address their needs, which enable the child to remain in the community, and do not require fitting the child and family into preexisting service models.

A therapeutic foster home, often called treatment foster care, delivers care in a private licensed home with specially trained foster parents who are considered professionals and who receive extensive pre-service training and in-service supervision and support (Chamberlain, 2000). Such foster homes typically take only one or two foster children. Wraparound and therapeutic foster homes are described in more detail in the final chapter of this book.

If available, a wraparound service model might have allowed Robert to remain with his mother and have provided the support that both of them needed. If out-of-home placement were necessary, a therapeutic foster home might have offered the structure and therapeutic intensity that Robert needed coupled with a nurturing environment. There is evidence that wraparound care and therapeutic foster care are able to serve children with quite severe emotional or behavioral problems (Berrick, Courtney, & Barth, 1993; Burchard, Burns, & Burchard, 2003; Chamberlain, 2000; Curtis, Alexander, & Lunghofer, 2001; Hudson, Nutter, & Gallaway, 1994). With none of these options available, Robert cycled in and out of the county emergency shelter, where he fared and behaved better than he did in other placement settings.

CASE STUDY OF ROBERT

Robert's parents knew each other from high school, but were never married nor had ever lived together. His mother's pregnancy with him was complicated. She had developed toxemia, an abnormal condition of pregnancy characterized by hypertension, tissue swelling, and high levels of protein in the urine. When Robert's mother, Cynthia, went into labor in her ninth month of pregnancy, she started having seizures. Her blood pressure remained high during her labor and delivery. Following his birth, Robert was required to remain in the hospital for two weeks because he too began having seizures.

Robert was always a difficult child for his mother to manage. When he was in preschool, he was found to have a limited attention span, uncooperative behavior, and an excessive tendency to fight with other children. Cynthia took him to see a psychiatrist at a county hospital when he was four, to help her deal with his hyperactivity and behavior problems. They saw the psychiatrist for about a year, but she continued having a hard time with Robert's behavior (see Exhibit 7.1).

EXHIBIT 7.1.
Placement History

Time Period	Placement	Maltreatment	School
Preschool	Parent Home		Preschool
1st Grade	Parent Home		Elem. School
			Stepping Stones NPS
2nd Grade	Parent Home		Stepping Stones NPS
3rd Grade	Parent Home		Stepping Stones NPS
4th Grade	Parent Home		Stepping Stones NPS
5th Grade	Parent Home	Abuse	Stepping Stones NPS
5th Grade	Langely Group Home		Kingston NPS

(continued)

(continued)

6th Grade	Parent Home		Stepping Stones NPS
	Hospital		Hospital School
	Parent Home	Abuse	Stepping Stones NPS
7th Grade	Shelter		Shelter School
	Hoffman RTP		Hoffman NPS
	Shelter		Shelter School
8th Grade	Shelter		Shelter School
9th Grade	Parent Home		Not in school
	Shelter		Shelter School
	Cavanaugh RTP		Cavanaugh NPS
	Emergency Shelter		Shelter School
10th Grade	Rockwood RTP		Rockwood NPS
	Shelter		Shelter School
	Baldwin Group Home		Gerard NPS
11th Grade	Baldwin Group Home		Gerard NPS
	Emergency Shelter		Shelter School
12th Grade	Helpful Bridge RTP		Helpful Bridge NPS
	Emergency Shelter		Shelter School
	Pine Tree RTP		Pine Tree NPS
	Emergency Shelter		Shelter School

Elem. = Elementary School.

NPS = Nonpublic School (i.e., a private special education school).

Elementary School Years

Robert started first grade when he was six. His teacher reported that, right from the first week of class, he showed stubbornness and, at times, very disruptive behavior. She felt he lacked self-control and, unless reprimanded strongly, he would walk around the classroom doing whatever he pleased. On several occasions, when he did not get his way, he threatened other children with the point of his pencil. His teacher observed that he had very rapid behavioral and mood changes.

Academically, Robert was far behind his peers. He was able to write his first name and a few numbers, but he demonstrated little progress toward retaining and applying newly taught material. The teacher felt he displayed excessive dependency on her for direction.

Within a month of starting first grade, the school nurse recommended to Robert's mother that she contact the Regional Center, an agency that provided services to children and adults with developmental disabilities. Cynthia promptly followed up on the nurse's suggestion. The Regional Center evaluated Robert, diagnosing him with attention deficit disorder with hyperactivity, suspected mental retardation, and a speech articulation disorder, possibly resulting from mental retardation. Because of his history of seizures, he was found to be eligible for Regional Center services, even though mental retardation was not clearly established (see Exhibit 7.2).

During the first-grade, Robert also became eligible for special education services on the basis of an emotional disturbance. He would retain this eligibility designation throughout his school years.

The individualized education program (IEP) team described Robert as engaging in a repetitive pattern of behavior in which the basic rights of others were violated. The teams' recommendation was for him to attend a nonpublic school, funded by the school district, because the district felt it could not adequately handle his difficult behaviors in its public school program. His mother placed him in Stepping Stones School, a nonpublic, state-certified school for children with learning and behavioral problems.

EXHIBIT 7.2.
Regional Center Eligibility

An individual is eligible for Regional Center services if, among other factors, he has one or more of the following conditions:

- Mental retardation
- Epilepsy
- Cerebral palsy
- Conditions found to be closely related to mental retardation
- Conditions requiring treatment similar to that required for mentally retarded individuals. (Lanterman Developmental Disabilities Act, 1969)

A neurology study done around this time suggested Robert had brain dysfunction consistent with partial seizures. Since he was continuing to have seizures on a fairly regular basis, he was placed on anticonvulsant medication.

During his elementary school years, Robert continued attending Stepping Stones School. In the second grade, the school staff struggled with his hyperactivity and short attention span, along with instances of unprovoked aggression, and a negative reaction to correction. Outside of a structured setting, without provocation, Robert would hit, kick, bite, and throw rocks at his peers.

During the second grade, Robert had two audiometric screenings. Both of them showed inconsistent scores for his right ear, varying from a moderate to profound hearing loss. However, no services were indicated nor classroom accommodations made to compensate for his hearing loss.

By the third grade, Robert was beginning to show somewhat better control of his aggressive impulses, which was attributed to the counseling he now was receiving at Stepping Stones; it was paid for by the school district. His peer relations had greatly improved and he was able to work cooperatively and attentively in a group setting. He still, however, was hyperactive and totally disorganized. He was constantly losing whatever possessions he had with him such as lunch money, paper, pencil, coat, or hat.

In addition, further testing of Robert's hearing indicated a moderate hearing loss in his right ear. Both his fine and gross motor skills were determined to be below his age and grade level. However, by the end of the third grade, Robert was able to read sight words at the beginning third grade level and his math skills were at the end of the second grade level. Both, his expressive and receptive, vocabulary were described as being severely limited and his syntax was poor. Consequently, the school district found him eligible to receive services from a language and speech specialist, once a week for thirty minutes, to address these language areas. However, no services were recommended to address his hearing loss.

In the fourth grade, Robert continued to be highly distractible and needed significant prompting from his teacher to stay on task. When he was frustrated, he would whine and he cried easily. There was concern expressed by the school psychologist and the nonpublic school staff that he had a poor grasp of reality, which included some paranoid aspects to his thinking.

Despite his difficulties, he continued to progress academically, particularly in reading and spelling. He also continued receiving weekly counseling and language and speech services.

What Had Gone Wrong?

While Robert was receiving counseling to address his emotional and behavioral problems and language and speech services to improve his below age and grade level language skills, he did not receive any services or classroom accommodations to address his hearing impairment. Once the hearing impairment had been identified, his IEP should have included strategies to address his needs in this area.

Advocacy Considerations

Robert's mother, or anyone else who was a member of his IEP team, could have asked at his IEP meeting for services and accommodations to address his hearing loss to be included on his IEP. If such services had been denied, then Robert's mother had the option of contesting this denial through the special education hearing process, which was used in Sharon's case as described in Chapter 2.

The First Petition Is Filed

Prevention

Robert first was removed from his mother's custody when he was in the fifth grade, after he had called the child protection services (CPS) hotline and reported that his mother had physically abused him. A petition then was filed alleging that she had inflicted multiple contusions to Robert's body. The allegations were sustained and Robert was declared a dependent of the juvenile court. He was removed from his mother's care and sent to the county emergency shelter. He then was placed in the Langely Group Home and started Kingston School, another nonpublic school.

Within six months, the court had terminated its jurisdiction in Robert's case and his mother's rights related to his care and custody were returned to her. Robert moved back in to his mother's home and starting attending Stepping Stones again, his old nonpublic school.

The school reports from Stepping Stones clearly indicate that the staff felt he had regressed emotionally in the six months he was in out-of-home placement and attending another school. He now was more timid and tearful. His initial response to correction was to begin whimpering. However, he was somewhat less aggressive and, when frustrated or angry, generally did not assault other children. Instead, he reacted by throwing his pencil or paper, shoving a desk or chair out of the way, or talking loudly using inappropriate language. He also had started demonstrating some unusual behaviors such as kissing his fingers, rocking in his chair, and laughing uproariously at odd times. During academic testing by the school psychologist, he did not maintain eye contact with her, and he talked frequently about earthquakes and that they would die in one, and then ran around grabbing and hugging her from behind.

On the positive side, Robert now was able to stay in his seat most of the time and keep his hands to himself. He could work on familiar tasks independently for periods of fifteen to twenty minutes at a time, and he usually raised his hand when seeking adult attention. His reading tested at the beginning fourth grade level and math at the beginning third grade level. On academic achievement tests, his strengths were in sight vocabulary, word attack skills, and spelling; weaknesses were in math application and language usage.

What Had Gone Wrong?

While the details of Robert's out-of-home placement are somewhat unclear, what is clear is that his behavior had deteriorated during the time he was removed from his mother's care. Since he only was out of his mother's home for six months, it raises the important question of whether Robert would have been better served by remaining in his mother's home, with intensive services provided to help his mother learn better parenting skills, rather than being placed away from her in a group home.

One of the major cracks in the child welfare system is that CPS agencies receive a large portion of their federal funding based on the number of abused or neglected children placed in out-of-home care (Adoption Assistance and Child Welfare Act [AACWA], 1980). There is significantly more federal funding available to support foster and adoptive families than birth parents, thus making it difficult for CPS agencies to provide preventive services prior to the removal of children from their parents' care (Reed & Karpilow, 2002). Some CPS agencies throughout the country have sought waivers to federal child welfare funding requirements to provide creative ways to deliver services, including in-home services to families (McCarthy et al., 2005; Reed & Karpilow, 2002). Obviously, the question of paramount importance is whether a child can remain safely in the home when intensive services are provided.

Back with His Mother

Robert started living with his mother again. He now was in the sixth grade.

Intervention

His mother followed up a Regional Center's referral for counseling. Six hours of counseling were provided for four months, and it was paid for by the Regional Center. Except for one two-hour session at Stepping Stones School, the remainder of the counseling sessions took place at Robert's home.

The purpose of the counseling was to improve Robert's socialization with his peers and decrease his temper tantrums and other inappropriate behavior. When Robert became angry, he pushed those around him or threw things at them. He also fought with peers, made inappropriate sexual and other comments to adults and peers, and could not be left alone unsupervised for even short periods of time without getting into serious trouble.

A positive behavior modification program was implemented where Robert received points for appropriate behavior. The daily points were tallied at the end of each week and traded for additional allowance money on the weekend. At the same time, inappropriate behavior did not earn Robert any points.

The behavior modification program implemented by the counselor was extremely effective with Robert. His temper tantrums were extinguished completely and his inappropriate way of interacting with others was significantly reduced. His mother felt, however, that she could not be consistent in marking points on a chart on an hourly basis, which was required in the original design of the program. Consequently, the program was modified. The counselor worked with Robert's mother to help her become more consistent and flexible in providing positive reinforcement and having more realistic expectations for Robert's behavior. She no longer removed all reinforcement opportunities for just one inappropriate behavioral incident.

During the course of Robert's counseling, he was evaluated by a psychiatrist and put on medication to reduce anxiety. The counselor working with him and his mother felt that the medication had a marked effect on Robert's ability to control his behavior and, in fact, made behavior modification a viable option for him. He still, however, could not safely be left alone unsupervised or when interacting with peers. On one occasion, when left home alone after school for a short period of time, he started a small fire in a trashcan. When his mother returned home and observed the charred paper in the trashcan, she confronted Robert. He said he was angry with her and, displaying considerable insight, told her he had burned the papers to show her how angry he was. The counselor recommended that Robert and his mother receive an additional three months of in-home counseling, for five hours each month. However, this additional counseling was not approved by the Regional Center, so it did not occur.

Some positive effects of the mental health treatment were seen in Robert's nonpublic school environment. He had an improved ability to express negative feelings without aggression or running away. But he continued to have difficulty verbalizing his feelings in a realistic manner. He would start off with a reality-based statement, but then embellish it to the point where a listener could not tell where the reality ended and the fantasy began. He still exhibited outbursts where he would whine or cry when corrected or knock over desks or throw things when angry. When working in a group setting, he would bring up topics that were off the subject, and tended to talk to himself rather than to others in the group.

The speech pathologist working with him noted that he really could not participate in a conversation. He was capable of initiating an interaction, securing permission to do something, and giving or getting information. But he could not maintain a topic of conversation over several utterances nor elaborate on a topic. The pathologist indicated that he would need training and support on how to verbally interact with others in various settings.

What Had Gone Wrong?

Since Robert had benefited significantly from the behavior modification program that a Regional Center counselor set up with his mother, this should have encouraged the Regional Center or CPS to ensure that counseling services be continued and that his mother receive ongoing support at the level she needed to maintain the positive modification program for her son. The fact these relatively inexpensive services were stopped, leading to the cycle of out-of-home placements that followed for Robert, has to be described as nothing less than a travesty and a severe crack in the system of protection and support for vulnerable families.

Psychiatric Hospitalization

Intervention

A little more than halfway through Robert's sixth-grade year, his mother started to find it more and more difficult to deal with his hyperactivity and aggressive behavior. She decided to place him in a hospital with a psychiatric unit for children. He remained there for five weeks. In the hospital, Robert's medication was evaluated and ultimately changed. In addition to anticonvulsant medication for his seizure disorder, he now started taking medication for a bipolar disorder (see Exhibit 7.3).

EXHIBIT 7.3.
Bipolar Disorder

Bipolar Disorder, also known as manic-depressive illness, is a serious medical illness that causes shifts in a person's mood, energy, and ability to function. Bipolar disorder causes dramatic mood swings from overly "high" and/or irritable to sad and hopeless, and then back again, often with periods of normal mood in between. Severe changes in energy and behavior go along with these changes in mood. (National Institute of Mental Health, n.d.)

On release from the hospital, Robert returned to his mother's home and to Stepping Stones, the nonpublic school he had been attending previously. Upon his return, the school noted that he now was more violent and aggressive than he previously had been. When he was angry, he would call his teachers and other students by derogatory names, and curse at them without apparent provocation. He knocked over desks and chairs and threw objects around the room during his tantrums. He vehemently would deny any responsibility for his explosive behavior. After he was back at Stepping Stones for about a month, the school staff said he started to gain better control of his behavior and the outbursts became less frequent. Even with all his problem behavior, Robert was continuing to progress in school academically.

What Had Gone Wrong?

Robert did not appear to have benefited from his five-week hospital stay. His mother placed him in the hospital right before his twelfth birthday. It is not clear whether the treatment itself was not adequate (including change of medication), or whether the aftercare was not sufficient, or whether his budding adolescence coupled with his mental health and family problems conspired to make it a very difficult time for him. It seems likely that a continuation of the in-home counseling and behavior modification program would have been more effective, both therapeutically and economically, than a five-week inpatient hospitalization.

Services Provided for the Hearing Impairment

Intervention

The school district finally identified Robert as being hard of hearing. He then started receiving services from an itinerant teacher for the deaf and hard-of-hearing to help him in auditory training, phonological skills, and speech reading.

Advocacy Considerations

Had Robert's mother been aware of her rights under special education law, she might have requested compensatory services for Robert for the time his hearing impairment first had been identified until the time he received services. Compensatory services are available under the IDEA (Assistance to States for the Education of Children with Disabilities, 2005), and in Robert's case, it might have included additional time from the itinerant teacher for the deaf and hard-of-hearing to make up for the service he should have had but did not receive.

Physical Abuse

At the beginning of summer, right around the time the school semester ended, Robert's mother called the police and reported that Robert had run away. She said this had occurred after she had spanked him. The police found Robert on a city bus. There were whip marks and broken skin on both of his arms. Robert told the police that his mother had hit him with a stick.

Prevention

The police took Robert into custody for his protection. He now was several months past his twelfth birthday.

What Had Gone Wrong?

Robert's mother, without the continued counseling services, had reverted to ineffective and illegal methods in trying to control her son's behavior.

Emergency Shelter

Prevention

Robert was sent to the county emergency shelter where, according to the staff, he had a difficult time adjusting. He had one of the staff members assigned to him full-time because he was not interacting appropriately with peers. In addition to behaving aggressively, he also was described as having a preoccupation with sex and engaging in inappropriate touching with staff.

A psychological evaluation completed at the time suggested that his mother's abuse of him and his extreme fear that she would kill him drove his aggression. He was diagnosed with posttraumatic stress disorder, borderline intellectual functioning, and a specific developmental disorder. The psychologist did not find Robert to be hyperactive, but he still was very distractible. Nevertheless, the psychologist reported that Robert was able to respond appropriately to direction. The psychologist made three recommendations for Robert's treatment: (1) he be placed in a mental health facility that provided structure and good behavior management, (2) he be referred for counseling since he responded well to the psychologist's interpretations of his feelings related to his past and present experiences, and (3) he be provided with special educational programming for a child with a learning disability.

Residential Treatment Facility

Intervention

After five months at the emergency shelter, Robert entered Hoffman, a therapeutic residential treatment program. Robert was in the seventh grade at this time. During the first month in this program, a staff psychologist completed a behavioral assessment of Robert and put together a positive behavior modification program for the purpose of changing his inappropriate behaviors. A referral also was made for a mental health assessment from the department of mental health (DMH) through the IEP process. The assessment completed by DMH, about four months after Robert entered the residential treatment program, showed that he still was having serious social and emotional problems. He had great difficulty in relating appropriately to both peers and adults. His socialization skills were described as extremely limited and he required a great deal of attention and prompting to help him act in socially appropriate ways. His frustration tolerance and impulse control were seen to be very low. In addition, he was unable to structure his own thinking process, often leading him to become aggressive. With signs of any lack of structure in his environment, he seemed to act out and become hostile.

DMH found that the Hoffman School, which was connected to the residential facility, did not provide an adequate therapeutic program to meet Robert's significant mental health needs. DMH consequently recommended and agreed to fund services from the facility's day treatment program, which offered individual therapy three times a week, group therapy twice a week, family therapy once a week, and medication monitoring twice a week. Robert also would continue to attend the Hoffman nonpublic school program.

Less than two months after the report by DMH, the clinical staff at the Hoffman residential program decided to discharge Robert. They expressed serious concerns about his level of physical aggression, which tended toward violence, ongoing property destruction, and inappropriate sexual behavior (i.e., exposing himself to others or using graphically sexual language). They described an incident where Robert had been calmly speaking with a female peer and then he became explosively angry in a flash of unprovoked rage. In the final analysis, he had engaged in four incidents, within a ten-day period, which led the staff to conclude that he required a different type of program. He had made homicidal threats to staff, became so physically aggressive that he required three men to restrain him, he also threatened a female counselor both physically and verbally, and was found unbuttoning the blouse of a young, frail, female student who was developmentally delayed, whom he had carried to the back of one of the facility's buildings. In addition, his mother reported, that while on an overnight home visit, he had either sexually molested or attempted to sexually molest a two-year-old child when, for a brief period for time, he was left unsupervised. The recommendation by the clinical staff of the Hoffman residential and day treatment program was that Robert required a program for adolescent sex-offenders. Robert now was thirteen and promptly was returned to the emergency shelter.

What Had Gone Wrong?

When Robert was hospitalized for five weeks during the sixth grade, one of his discharge diagnoses had been bipolar disorder. The bipolar diagnosis, subsequently, seems to have disappeared from psychiatric or psychological assessments of him. Clearly, those assessing and treating Robert should have been aware of this diagnosis and considered whether his behaviors were related to a bipolar disorder, warranting specific medications for their control.

A Permanency Planning Hearing

Up until this point, Robert's case plan had stated that family reunification was the goal for Robert and his mother. At a court hearing held shortly after Robert was returned to the emergency shelter, the goal now was changed from family reunification to long-term out-of home placement. The reason given for this change was that Robert's complex problems required special programs and, in spite of his mother's good intentions, they exceeded her ability to meet his needs. She was required to visit him on a regular basis and participate in his treatment. Her cooperation with the past plan had been judged satisfactory.

Shortly after this hearing, Nancy, senior attorney at Advocacy Services, was appointed to represent Robert. She was appointed in this case because of her expertise in working with multiple agencies to attain services for difficult-to-place children.

Attempting to Locate an Appropriate Placement

At the next court hearing, held just twenty-one days after the previous hearing, the judge indicated, and put in the court report, that an interagency effort was required to identify an appropriate program to meet Robert's needs. The agencies involved in this joint effort, which already had started working on his case, were special CPS and DMH placement units and the Regional Center. Also included in this court report were a referral for a new psychological evaluation of Robert and a recommendation to refer him for admission to Moreno State Hospital. The psychologist and psychiatric social worker from the DMH placement unit made the state hospital recommendation believing that Robert should be placed with individuals with developmental disabilities who could not live safely in the community.

Following the court hearing, the Regional Center submitted a packet of information about Robert to Moreno State Hospital and, in addition, began a statewide search to find other programs deemed appropriate. Sometime after, Nancy contacted Robert's Regional Center worker and learned that the state hospital had rejected admitting him, stating that his behavior did not warrant placement in a locked state hospital program. Furthermore, a Moreno State Hospital staff member had conveyed that, based on Robert's previous psychological evaluations, he did not appear to have mental retardation, which was a necessary criterion for admission. Rather, this staff person said, according to the evaluation reports, he primarily had a serious emotional disturbance and only borderline mental retardation. Also expressed was the concern that Robert would attack other children in the program who had significant developmental delays.

Another bit of information conveyed by the Regional Center worker was that she had contacted the adolescent sex-offender program at Moreno State Hospital and was told Robert would be accepted in that program only if a Superior Court ordered it on the basis of him being a danger to himself or others. Robert's behavior, at that time, did not appear to rise to the level of satisfying that legal criterion.

Advocacy Considerations

State law clearly specified that no mentally retarded person may be committed to the state hospital unless a finding is made by the Superior Court that he or she is a danger to himself/herself or others (Admissions & Judicial Commitments, 2001). Danger to self or others, under this provision of state law, included, but was not limited to, a finding of incompetence to stand trial, having been charged with a murder or mayhem, inflicting great bodily injury to another, robbery perpetrated by torture or by a person armed with a dangerous or deadly weapon, among other conditions. Although Robert's aggressive behavior often was difficult to contain and sometimes injurious to others, it did not seem to meet standard of the danger to self or others.

Regional Center Denies Eligibility

The psychologist who provided the court-ordered evaluation of Robert reported that he found no evidence of his having mental retardation. It was the psychologist's opinion that Robert's significant emotional disturbance compromised his ability to show his true intellectual potential. During the course of the evaluation, Robert had gone into explicit detail about having had sex with his girlfriend and having discussed with his six- and nine-year-old cousins the mechanics of having a baby. Based on this discussion, the psychologist was of the decided opinion that the sophistication of his communication, including his sexual descriptions, far exceeded what one would expect of an individual with mental retardation.

An unintended consequence of this evaluation was that the Regional Center decided to review Robert's eligibility for the agency's services and found "he did not have a developmental disability diagnosis." As a result, the Regional Center concluded he no longer was eligible for the services.

Nancy appealed the denial of eligibility for Robert on the grounds that he, contrary to the Regional Center's position, in fact, qualified for services based on the broader federal definition of developmental disability (Developmental Disability Act, 1984). In keeping with its procedures, the Regional Center then reviewed Robert's eligibility for services again. This time the Regional Center reversed its position and decided to reinstate Robert's eligibility (see Exhibit 7.4).

EXHIBIT 7.4.
Federal Definition of Developmental Disability

The term "developmental disability" means a severe, chronic disability of an individual that

A. is attributable to a mental or physical impairment or combination of mental and physical impairment
B. is manifested before the individual attains age twenty-two
C. is likely to continue indefinitely
D. results in substantial functional limitations in three or more of the following areas of major life activity:
  i. self-care;
  ii. receptive and expressive language;
  iii. learning;
  iv. mobility;
  v. self-direction;
  vi. capacity for independent living; and
  vii. economic self-sufficiency; and
E. reflects the individual's need for a combination and sequence of special, interdisciplinary, or generic services, individualized supports, or other forms of assistance that are of lifelong or extended duration and are individually planned and coordinated.

An individual from birth to age nine, inclusive, who has substantial developmental delay or specific congenital or acquired conditions may be considered to have a developmental disability without meeting three or more of the criteria described above in (A) through (E) if the individual, without services and supports, has a high probability of meeting those criteria later in life. (Developmental Disabilities Act, 1984, §6001(7))

Regional Center Again Denies Eligibility

Almost a year later, the Regional Center again questioned Robert's eligibility for services and again denied that he qualified for them. Nancy, consequently, once more appealed the eligibility denial decision, which led to a review by a Regional Center multidisciplinary team. This time, however, the review team did not reinstate his eligibility based on the broader federal definition. Therefore, Nancy appealed the denial of eligibility by the multidisciplinary team and was prepared to argue the case at a state-level administrative hearing (Lanterman Developmental Disabilities Services Act, 1969). Prior to the hearing, Pam, the Advocacy Services staff attorney, continued to negotiate with the Regional Center assistant director, which ultimately proved to be a good strategy. Not long before the hearing date, the assistant director sent a letter to Pam stating that the Regional Center would reinstate eligibility for Robert. The rationale given was that Robert had required and received services similar to those provided to persons diagnosed with a developmental disability. Since he had been found eligible in the past and furthermore, since his condition had not significantly improved, it would be difficult, the assistant director wrote, to justify the denial of continued eligibility.

Advocacy Considerations

Three main advocacy strategies were used to maintain Regional Center eligibility for Robert. First, it was the use and understanding of the Regional Center appeal procedures. Second, it was the importance of knowing in detail both the state law, on which the Regional Center based its eligibility decisions, and also the federal law, which set the standard for what constituted a developmental disability. Third, it was keeping communication open and continuing to try to negotiate the desired outcome while still maintaining pressure on the Regional Center by having a hearing date scheduled.

Home with Mom

While the negotiations were going on over whether Robert qualified for Regional Center eligibility, the Regional Center continued to try to locate a residential treatment facility that was appropriate for him. A few programs, which the Regional Center contacted, agreed to review packets of information about him, but ultimately turned down his admission to their programs. Finally, Cavanaugh, a residential facility specifically for individuals with developmental disabilities expressed an interest in admitting him, but wanted to monitor his behavior before making a decision. However, Cavanaugh did not have an immediate opening.

At this point, Robert had been residing at the emergency shelter for about a year and had been doing fairly well. His aggressive behavior and inappropriate social interaction had greatly diminished. He also had been spending weekends at home with his mother without any serious behavioral incidents. Given that there were no immediate permanent placement options for Robert, CPS discussed with his mother the possibility of him living with her again.

Nancy had serious concerns about Robert being placed back in his mother's home. Although his behavior had improved significantly at the emergency shelter, he still required enormous time and the efforts of numerous staff members to keep his behavior contained. Nancy discussed her reservations with his mother and also his CPS caseworker. Nevertheless, Robert was sent home for a sixty-day trial visit during the summer.

Intervention

In order to help make this trial home visit work, Nancy requested respite services from the Regional Center, so Robert's mother would be able to have some time away from him while someone else was looking after him (see Exhibit 7.5).

EXHIBIT 7.5.
Respite Services

Respite services provide a break from caring for a child with a disability. Trained parents or others with training or expertise take care of the child for a brief period of time to give families relief from the strain of caring for the child. Respite services may be provided in the home or in another location. Some parents may require this help every week.

At the end of sixty days, Robert's mother reported that the situation with Robert at home was going fairly well, so the court changed the home-placement order from a trial basis to a permanent home-of parent placement. Within a very short time after that, however, Robert's mother called the CPS worker demanding that Robert immediately be removed from her home. She told the worker that Robert had refused to obey her and that she was afraid of him.

What Had Gone Wrong?

Robert had been placed with his mother during the summer. This was a time when he was out of school and not involved in any structured activities. Other than the small amount of respite time his mother received from the Regional Center, she had to be with him constantly. By the time she felt that she no longer could handle him at home, Robert had been out of school for almost four months. It frankly did not make sense for CPS to place Robert with his mother without also putting in place the services and activities that would have made a likely successful placement.

Robert's CPS caseworker had her own perspective on why the placement with his mother failed. She felt that the problem arose because of Robert's mother's inability to make a commitment to him and, consequently, she became increasingly anxious about having him in her custody. Furthermore, she believed that his mother was unprepared emotionally to deal with him, and his escalating acting out behavior was perhaps a reaction to her own ambivalence. If the social worker was right about why Robert's placement with his mother did not work out, it clearly seems that CPS was negligent in placing him with her without any services in place to try to improve the likelihood that the placement would be successful. Implementing a home-of-parent placement without any serious planning or having support services in place indicates a major crack in the child welfare placement process (see Exhibit 7.6).

Placement at a Residential Facility

Intervention

Robert returned to the emergency shelter and a month later to Cavanaugh, the residential treatment facility that had been considering

**EXHIBIT 7.6.
Placement Planning**

When placing a child with serious emotional and behavioral problems in the home of his parent, ensure that all necessary services are in place to support the placement.

accepting him, which had an opening and decided to admit him. Cavanaugh was in another county, in an idyllic, natural setting. All of the individuals, that is, children and adults, at Cavanaugh had developmental disabilities. Many had a significant degree of mental retardation. There was a small program for those who had both a developmental disability and also significant emotional and behavioral problems.

Robert only lasted four months at Cavanaugh before being discharged. According to Robert's CPS caseworker, his behavior in this program was marginal from the beginning. He had been caught trying to "overpower" a couple of girls at the Cavanaugh facility, but was stopped by staff before anything happened. Then three weeks before he was discharged, he, along with another resident, was using gang signs, which provoked a fight and reportedly incited a riot. Robert ended up hitting one of his counselors.

The Cavanaugh staff had Robert arrested and he was placed on informal probation. The facility administrator then gave CPS a notice that he wanted Robert removed immediately. The CPS social worker, however, refused to go and pick him up believing he was not safe to transport. Finally, Cavanaugh sent one of its staff members to transport Robert back to the emergency shelter, after giving him a major tranquilizer.

What Had Gone Wrong?

In some ways, it was surprising that Cavanaugh accepted Robert in the first place since the facility had a reputation of not having much tolerance for residents with a propensity for aggressive or sexually acting out behavior. Consequently, there was not really an appropriate program in place to deal with these behaviors.

When Robert entered the Cavanaugh residential program, his mother was unable to visit him because its location was more than a three-hour drive from her home. This may also have negatively affected Robert's behavior. Clearly, CPS should have made arrangements to enable Robert to see his mother on a regular basis during this period of time.

Cycling in an Out of the Emergency Shelter

Intervention

Robert returned to the emergency shelter where he remained for four months before being placed at yet another residential treatment facility, called Rockwood. He remained at Rockwood for only twenty days before being sent back to the emergency shelter because of his aggressive behavior. Robert still clung to the idea of living with his mother again.

Robert's IEP during this time indicated that he still had deficits in pragmatic language skills and difficulty interpreting social situations. He continued to have inappropriate behavior when relating to peers and adults, including making sexual remarks and engaging in inappropriate physical contact. However, he was not running away or vandalizing property. His mother was visiting him regularly and was interested in receiving family counseling. He also was having successful home visits again.

Group Home Placement Fails to Supervise Robert

Intervention

This time Robert remained at the emergency shelter for nine months. Then he was placed in the Baldwin Group Home, a six-bed home for adolescent males. Initially, he had a positive adjustment to this group home and also to the individual counseling. His mother remained active in his life, visiting him twice a month, and he had occasional overnight home visits. As time went on, however, Robert's behavior began to deteriorate and he became more and more out of control. He choked another resident, broke windows, and destroyed other property of the Baldwin Group Home.

About the same time, his mother became seriously concerned that Robert was not being supervised adequately at this group home. When driving about ten miles from the home, she came across Robert wandering aimlessly on the street. He was dirty and unkempt. Robert reported to his mother that a staff person at the group home hit him on the head with a paddle.

When Pam, the Advocacy Services staff attorney, called the Baldwin Group Home to discuss the supervision issue, she was promptly informed that Robert had been "caught masturbating" in his own room at the home. Consequently, five months after Robert had first been placed in this group home he was removed by mutual consent of all parties involved and returned once more to the emergency shelter. Robert had just turned sixteen at the time.

What Had Gone Wrong?

It not only appears that this placement did not have an appropriate treatment program for Robert, but it also failed to provide necessary supervision.

Advocacy Consideration

One of the issues that we at Advocacy Services discussed was whether the group home staff should have been so ready to discharge Robert because of his masturbating in the privacy of his room. Clearly, no one at the office condoned sexual behavior that inappropriately involved or was harmful to others. We also were aware of Robert's history of inappropriate sexual remarks and touching. However, the issue of individuals with disabilities being able to engage in appropriate sexual behavior while living in a group care setting has been raised as a serious issue by disability advocates (Hingsburger & Tough, 2002). We also wondered, at times, but had no way of knowing whether the fact that Robert was a large African-American male made his sexual remarks or actions seem more threatening to white treatment staff.

Assessment at a New Residential Treatment Facility

Robert once again returned to the emergency shelter. We, at Advocacy Services, become aware that a new residential treatment facility,

Helpful Bridge, had opened in an adjoining county for youngsters with brain injuries. This facility had a multidisciplinary treatment team and a structured program. Pam spent considerable time contacting the new program to discuss whether Robert would be an appropriate resident. Because of Pam's efforts, Robert was accepted at Helpful Bridge for a thirty-day assessment. After the assessment period, the program staff would determine Robert's appropriateness for the program.

The assessment completed by the treatment team found that Robert was functioning academically between the fifth and the tenth-grade levels. His letter-word identification score put him at the end of the tenth grade level in this skill area. Math calculation was at the beginning of the seventh grade. His lowest academic score was on his writing sample, which was evaluated at the beginning of the fifth grade. Robert's speech and language assessment revealed that his receptive and expressive language skills were at the eleven-year-old level, rather than equivalent to his age of sixteen and a half.

At the end of the thirty-day assessment period, when the treatment team was considering whether Robert was an appropriate candidate for this residential program, he became sexually involved with a young, female student at the facility, ensuring he would be terminated from the program. What happened was that one evening, when Robert had just returned from an outing with a staff member and a few other residents, he was found, during a routine room check, in the bathroom with a twelve-year-old female resident. They were both lying on the floor. The girl was naked and lying on her back. Robert was lying on his side with his pants down. The staff member immediately returned Robert to his own room and he was kept under continuous visual surveillance.

When interviewed by the psychologist at the facility, Robert relayed that he had become friendly with the girl and had let her listen to his musical tapes. He claimed that she told him, "I like you, you're cute," and he replied, "I like you too, but chill out . . . it isn't going to be like that." Robert said he didn't know how old she was, but thought she was older than twelve years.

Robert claimed that when he had returned from the outing, the girl knocked on her window from inside her room and then opened the door for him. He said, once he was in her room, they started kissing, and she took him into the bathroom. Robert reported that he was "kissing her by her belly button" when they were caught. He claimed that "there was no touching anywhere else" and that he did not have an erection and didn't know why it was such a big deal.

One of the major concerns of the psychologist, other than the fact that the incident had occurred at all, was that Robert did not express remorse or concern about what had happened. He did not acknowledge any repercussions for the girl and seemed to have no understanding of any obligation to have avoided her on the evening of the incident. Consequently, the psychologist was of the opinion that Robert was not appropriate for the Helpful Bridge program because he lacked the judgment or ability to conform to the facility's norms and rules. Furthermore, he was impulsive and insensitive to others or their feelings, which suggested to the psychologist a developing antisocial personality disorder. He felt that Robert's most salient difficulties were those of a mental health nature rather than those of a typical youth with brain injuries. It was the psychologist's opinion that Robert should reside in a setting with more safeguards and mental health services than that facility could provide.

What Had Gone Wrong?

Helpful Bridge had accepted Robert with full knowledge of his past behavior. At the time, however, the facility was new and had many available beds. By the time Robert was discharged, the facility was full and had a waiting list. At that point, the staff was concerned about the facility's liability.

Nevertheless, Robert may not have been appropriate for this program. It seems that his lack of judgment or inability to control his sexual behavior was not something for which this program was designed. The difficult question, however, was where a program that was designed to meet Robert's tremendous needs could be found?

Final Attempt at Residential Treatment Facility Placement

Robert was returned to the emergency shelter. After a three-month stay, Robert once again was placed in another residential treatment facility. This facility, called Pine Tree, had full knowledge of the incident involving the twelve-year-old girl that had led to Robert's discharge from Helpful Bridge and the other inappropriate sexual behavior he had engaged in over the years.

During the intake psychiatric evaluation at Pine Tree, Robert's mood was described as depressed and angry and he exhibited guardedness, passive defiance, and possible paranoia. He described himself as ruthless and mean. When asked by the psychiatrist who he looked up to, he reported that he did not have anyone he looked up to except for himself. The psychiatrist concluded that Robert had some potential for verbal abstract reasoning but his judgment was impaired due to a history of poor impulse control and he possessed very limited insight into his problems.

During Robert's placement at Pine Tree, Pam kept in regular contact with the treatment staff. There was considerable concern expressed about Robert's aggressive outbursts toward peers. The staff felt there was no particular incident precipitating Robert's hostile, aggressive behavior, but that he would just "go off" about two or three times a week. About once a week, the behavior reached a level of dangerousness requiring the use of five-point restraints. In order to try to reduce Robert's aggressive outbursts, he was put on medication. He also was on a behavior modification program with frequent positive reinforcement.

The treatment staff reported that Robert was emotionally needy and wanted to be hugged frequently. However, he also engaged in inappropriate sexual touching with girls and boys about two or three times a week, in addition to making frequent, inappropriate sexual comments.

After four months in the Pine Tree program, Robert's CPS worker was given notice that Robert was being discharged from the facility. On the discharge summary, Robert's case manager at the facility indicated that he had made little improvement in his behavior during his stay there. He remained prone to explosive temper outbursts accompanied by physical aggression toward peers or staff, one to two times per week. He also would engage in inappropriate touching of peers almost daily. During his last month at the facility, he was unable to keep a roommate because of his threats of sexual assault and inappropriate touching of others. Not surprisingly, his behaviors were found to have detrimental effect both in the residential unit and at the school, causing an increase in the anxiety level of his peers.

After notice was given of Robert's discharge but before he actually was removed from Pine Tree, he became combative, and threatened to kill himself and harm the Pine Tree staff. Consequently, Robert was hospitalized involuntarily for being a danger both to himself and to others. He remained in the hospital for five days and then was transferred to the emergency shelter. In the short time that Robert was hospitalized, he exhibited a dramatic decrease in his combative behavior and an increase in his ability to tolerate limits. At discharge, he was bright and cheerful and denied any plan or intent to harm himself or anyone else.

Living at the Emergency Shelter

Within a week of Robert's return to the emergency shelter, there was an IEP meeting held. Pam learned at the meeting that Robert had been assigned a one-on-one aide that was with him at all times while at the emergency shelter. Robert's teachers strongly expressed their views that he needed the one-on-one, even when in their classes, because they perceived a change in his personality. They felt, since he had returned from the Pine Tree residential program, he was more aggressive and easier to set off than previously.

A little over a month after Robert had returned to the emergency shelter, Pam received a report that he was doing quite well there. He had not had any explosive outbursts or incidents of aggression. He still had his one-to-one aide with him at all times and, although he said he really did not like having the aide, he had not rebelled against it.

Around this time, Pam learned that the CPS special placement unit and DMH, once again, were considering filing the special petition that was required to have Robert placed in a state hospital. They had gone back to their original plan of placing him at Moreno State Hospital, in the unit for individuals with mental retardation. Pam, in discussions with the special placement unit staff, argued, as she had in the past, that Robert did not meet the criteria for involuntary placement. These arguments again prevailed in keeping Robert out of the state hospital.

The question that remained, however, was where Robert would live. He was about to turn eighteen and was very unrealistic about the future. He also was quite depressed about its uncertainty. Pam decided to call a meeting at the emergency shelter with Robert's CPS case-worker and other relevant agency personnel to discuss his long-term placement options. For the time being, Robert would live at the emergency shelter. The overriding question, however, was where would Robert live in the future when CPS no longer was responsible for him and he, therefore, could not remain at the emergency shelter.

At the meeting, Robert's Regional Center caseworker agreed to initiate a search, both countywide and statewide, to try to identify a place for Robert to live once he became an adult. Pam agreed to try to find adult transition services for Robert, to help him learn to live in the community as independently as possible.

After the meeting, the Regional Center worker initiated a county-wide search for adult-assisted living facilities for Robert, which did not initially turn up any facilities that agreed to interview him. Pam contacted an agency that provided transition services, but was told that Robert did not qualify for them because, at that time, he still was living at the emergency shelter and, therefore, not living independently. When Robert turned eighteen, the county agreed to continue providing funding for him until an appropriate community facility was found that would take him.

CONCLUSION

Robert was a young man who had tremendous needs that could not be met with the group home or residential treatment options available to him. Advocacy Services attorneys struggled with finding placement alternatives that would be in Robert's best interests. It was almost an impossible task.

Questions remain about whether he had an untreated bipolar disorder that brought on his rage, paranoia, and perhaps compulsive sexual behavior. There also are questions about whether his developmental disability ever was adequately understood so that appropriate strategies could have been developed to deal with his genuine areas of limitation. Although he was quite verbal, time and again he was assessed with both expressive and receptive language delays. His cognitive functioning level was in the area described as borderline, hovering somewhere between the upper end of mild mental retardation and the lower end of average. Assessments revealed that he had limited insight, abstract-reasoning deficits, and auditory memory problems. On top of that, he had a hearing loss, which likely affected his understanding of situations.

Robert was deemed too sophisticated for residential programs that catered to individuals with mental retardation. However, his seemingly unprovoked aggressive behavior, coupled with his limited insight, turned out to be beyond what most mental health residential programs could handle, particularly as he grew older and larger. The single deterrent, however, to his placement stability as he became an adolescent was his sexual behavior. He did not know either what was appropriate and inappropriate sexual behavior or did not have the impulse control to limit his own actions. None of the facilities where he was living had a program in place to deal with this issue (Ward & Bosek, 2002).

Given the options available, designing a program for Robert at the emergency shelter, which took his needs into account better than other settings, seemed appropriate. He was reasonably content at the emergency shelter and his behavior was more in control. The shelter had DMH staff on site who were able to monitor his mental health and medication needs. While Robert remained in the shelter, Pam was able to marshal the resources of the four agencies responsible for his care—CPS, DMH, the Regional Center, and the school—and work on transition goals and begin to plan for when he would "age out" of the foster care system.

SUMMARY

The purpose of this chapter primarily was: (1) to describe the problems that occur when in-home services provided for a mother and son are not sufficiently intensive, and, furthermore, when they are stopped prematurely; (2) to delineate the difficulty in finding an appropriate out-of-home placement for a youth whose mental health problems are not well understood and when they include inappropriate sexual behavior; and (3) to show how a creative solution was required to bring about placement stability for Robert and begin a transition process to ready him for a time when he no longer would be in the foster care system.

Chapter 8

Debra:
Supplementing the Appropriate Program

INTRODUCTION

For some foster youths who have unique needs, finding and maintaining an appropriate placement for them requires interagency collaboration and coordination. Child protective services (CPS) may need to work closely with agencies that deliver services to individuals with mental retardation or psychiatric disorders. CPS also may need to employ creative ways to fund programs and services for difficult-to place youth.

The case of Debra, an African-American female, who was diagnosed as having mental retardation, had trouble being maintained in a stable living situation. She also had trouble enrolling in a school program when she was placed in a foster home in the summer. The school district, where the foster home was located, was small. It did not have an appropriate classroom for her and had few special education staff working in the summer months.

Debra ultimately required the services of the Regional Center, an agency that procures services for those with developmental disabilities, in order to find her an appropriate group home with a public school program nearby. However, since this group home only served individuals with mental retardation, it could not deal fully with Debra's psychiatric disorder-related difficult behaviors. The question for Advocacy Services then became whether the group home could be supplemented in some way to make it an appropriate program for

doi:10.1300/5136_08

Debra and, furthermore, enable the staff to not become "burnt out" dealing with her on a daily basis.

This chapter details not only Debra's history leading up to placement in this group home, but also the advocacy efforts needed upon placement, for CPS to continue paying for the placement and to supplement the program so that Debra could remain there. Debra's case is an example of the kinds of efforts needed to create placement stability in the lives of some foster youths.

CASE STUDY OF DEBRA

Not much is known of Debra's birth history and early years. She was abandoned when she was eleven. Janet, the woman who Debra claimed had adopted her (although no adoption records ever were found) and with whom she was living at the time she was abandoned, left her with a "babysitter," and never returned. The babysitter later reported to CPS that Janet had told her she had adopted Debra as a baby and that Debra's biological mother, Penny, had mental retardation, thus making it easy for Janet to adopt Debra.

When the babysitter realized that Janet was not returning to retrieve Debra, she promptly called CPS. Debra then was taken by a social worker to the emergency shelter, where she was detained.

Debra claimed that Janet had once owned a house, which, for reasons not quite clear, she had lost. According to Debra, her adoptive mother and a male friend then moved them into a downtown hotel and Debra stopped attending school. When her mother was unable to pay her share of the hotel room because, according to Debra, she was smoking dope all day, the male friend kicked them out and they ended up living in cars and on the street. It was at this point, presumably, that Janet left her at the babysitter's and failed to retrieve her.

The babysitter relayed that she did not know Janet very well when she left Debra with her. She said she had seen her over several months in the neighborhood. She did know, however, and told CPS that Janet only was able to cash her welfare check at one check-cashing establishment in the area because she had no identification. CPS never was able to locate either Debra's adoptive or biological mother.

The Petition

The petition to the juvenile court alleged that Debra's mother left her with an unrelated caretaker without making a plan for her care and supervision. The petition was sustained during the adjudication hearing and Debra became a dependent of the juvenile court.

Prevention

At the time CPS initially picked up Debra from Janet's home, she was taken and detained at the emergency shelter. She attended the on-grounds school at the shelter in a special education class and received language and speech services and psychological counseling. During Debra's stay at the emergency shelter, the school psychologist estimated her cognitive level, and also how she interacted with others, to be like a much younger child of two to four years of age. Debra was twelve at the time (see Exhibit 8.1).

Group Home Placements

Debra's first placement was in a six-bed group home called Maybelle. Her stay at Maybelle was short. When the staff at Maybelle could no longer handle her behavior, she was switched to the Abilene Group Home, which also had six beds. Neither of these group homes worked out, however. Debra's behavior became uncontrollable and too difficult for the staff to manage. When she was discharged from the second group home, Debra's social worker described her as being overmedicated. She seemed like she was drugged. The social worker took Debra back to the emergency shelter.

What Had Gone Wrong?

The fact that Debra seemed overmedicated when her social worker retrieved her from the Abilene Group Home is a fairly good indication that this group home was not equipped to deal with her behavior. It also raises the question of whether her medication was being monitored sufficiently.

EXHIBIT 8.1.
Placement History Overview

Time Period	Placement	Maltreatment	School
Birth-11 yrs.	Parent (Biol./Adopt.)	Abandonment	N/A
12yrs.	Emergency Shelter		Shelter School
	Maybelle Grp. Home		Apollo School
	Abilene Grp. Home		Apollo School
	Emergency Shelter		Shelter School
	Foster Parent		N/A
	Emergency Shelter		Shelter School
	Foster Parent		Not in school
	Psychiatric Hospital		N/A
	Shelter		Shelter School
	Foster Parent		Lincoln Jr. High
13 yrs	Foster Parent		Lincoln Jr. High
	Shelter		Shelter School
14 yrs	Cavanaugh RTP		Cavanaugh NPS
	Psychiatric Hospital		N/A
	Cavanaugh RTP		Cavanaugh NPS
	Psychiatric Hospital		N/A
	Emergency Shelter		Shelter School
14 yrs 9 mos.	Gardner Group Home		Markham High

N/A = No records available.

Jr. High = Junior High or Middle School.

NPS = Nonpublic School (i.e., a private special education school).

High = High School.

School Placement

Intervention

During her time in the group homes, Debra attended the Apollo Program, a county-run special education program for children with severe emotional disturbance. She was in a full-day special education classroom and received counseling weekly for a twenty to thirty minute session. She also had a one-on-one behavior-management assistant with her full time at school. Those who worked with Debra in this program described her as functioning like a child who had both a severe emotional disturbance and mild mental retardation.

Advocacy Services Appointed

Debra was living at the emergency shelter when Nancy, Advocacy Services' senior attorney, was appointed to represent her. In Nancy's first conversation with Debra, Debra told her that she had tried to jump from a second-storey window at the Abilene Group Home because she had not been given enough food. Nancy emphasized to Debra that if she encountered future problems in her placements, she should contact Nancy because it was Nancy's job to take care of those kinds of problems for her.

After her visit with Debra, Nancy thoroughly reviewed Debra's juvenile court file to try to get a better picture of who her new client was. A recently completed psychological evaluation placed Debra at the low end of the mild mental retardation range. However, the psychologist who tested her felt that if Debra's hyperactivity were better controlled she might have scored somewhat higher on the intelligence test, but still not high enough to put her within the normal range of intelligence. While the psychologist reported that Debra had some basic self-help skills, like feeding herself and using the toilet, he also felt that she was substantially disabled in a wide range of areas, such as her ability to learn, engage in self-care and self-direction, and in her capacity for independence and self-sufficiency. Her academic skills were only at the preschool level. He also was of the opinion that her emotional functioning was marginal. He determined that although she did not have an acute psychosis, there was a histrionic quality to her behavior. Because she was so hyperactive and had poor judgment, and also behaved impulsively, the psychologist recommended that she be placed in a residential treatment facility with a highly structured environment (rather than in a foster or group home). He particularly felt that she needed a setting that was able to provide appropriate and immediate feedback to her about her behavior.

Foster Home Placement

Intervention

Despite the recommendation of the psychologist for Debra to be placed in a residential treatment facility, the day after Nancy visited Debra, she was placed on a trial basis in the home of Maryanne, a foster parent in whom the social worker had great confidence. The social worker described Maryanne to Nancy as a very special foster mother and told Nancy that she believed the placement would be successful.

The social worker was woefully mistaken. This foster home placement lasted only one night and day before Maryanne called the social worker to have Debra removed from her home. She told the social worker that the trial placement had been a total failure and that Debra had become destructive and suicidal.

Debra was returned to the emergency shelter again and this time classified as a "hard-to-place minor." This classification allowed the emergency shelter's Special Placement Unit to become involved in helping to find a new placement for her.

What Had Gone Wrong?

The psychologist who had evaluated Debra recommended that she be placed in a residential facility with a highly structured program. CPS did not take the evaluator's advice against placing her in a traditional foster home, even one with a highly regarded foster parent. This foster parent did not have the training, support, or structure in her home to address Debra's needs.

Yet Another Foster Home

Intervention

About a month later, Debra was placed in the home of another foster parent, Lucille. It was in the beginning of July when this placement occurred. Advocacy Services had law student interns working in the office in the summer and one of them, Carol, started assisting Nancy on Debra's case. Carol put in a call to Lucille and learned that Debra was, to put it mildly, quite a handful for her. Lucille relayed to Carol an incident, which she described as fairly minor, where Debra assaulted one of the home's hired staff members who was helping care for the children. Although Debra could be quite difficult, Lucille told Carol she wanted to continue caring for her. She thought that with the new medication that had been prescribed and more focused attention, which she intended to provide to Debra herself, Debra would be able to remain in her home.

Regional Center Denial

When Advocacy Services started representing Debra, Nancy realized that no one ever had applied for services for her from the Regional Center, the agency within the state set up to provide services for individuals with developmental disabilities. Consequently, at one of the first juvenile court hearings that Nancy attended as Debra's appointed attorney, she asked the court to order CPS to make a referral for eligibility for Debra to the Regional Center, which the court immediately did.

CPS then followed through with this court order and submitted an application for Debra to the Regional Center. Carol called the Regional Center to follow up on the application. She spoke to the counselor handling Debra's case. The counselor indicated that the case was under review, but she thought it was doubtful that Debra would be found eligible for services. The reason for this, she relayed, was that Debra's low functioning was due to a psychiatric disorder rather than mental retardation.

Carol called the Regional Center counselor back about a week later. She learned that a definite decision had been made and that Debra was found ineligible for Regional Center services. A letter from the Regional Center confirming the denial of eligibility arrived a few days later.

Contesting Regional Center Denial of Eligibility

Nancy filed for a state-level hearing to contest the denial of Regional Center Services for Debra, which led to an informal meeting, the first step in the appeal process. At the informal meeting, Nancy presented the case to the Regional Center administrator and the other professional staff present as to why Debra, in fact, did meet the Regional Center eligibility requirements and, therefore, should be made eligible for services. She argued that Debra's low functioning was not solely the result of her psychiatric disorder, but rather primarily caused by her developmental disability. She used the available assessment reports on Debra to substantiate her position (see Exhibit 8.2).

After the informal meeting, a written notification of the decision was supposed to arrive within five days, according to state law (Lanterman Developmental Disabilities Services Act, 1969). In this case, however, the Regional Center staff decided they wanted additional time for a mental health work up of Debra before making their decision as to her eligibility.

Enrollment in School

Debra had been placed in Lucille's home during the summer. Lucille wanted to enroll Debra in a school program as soon as possible, so that she would have a structured program during the day to help her move ahead academically and also she would be settled in an appropriate school program by the fall. However, the school district in which Lucille's home was located was fairly small and, as it turned out, most of the special education teachers, administrators, and school psychologists were off for the summer months. Not realizing that she would run into a problem, Lucille called the school district intending to enroll Debra, but could not get anyone in the district to even talk with her.

Nancy decided to contact the school district to see if she could make some headway in enrolling Debra in school. While she was not successful in enrolling her in a school program that summer, she learned that it was unlikely the district had an appropriate program for Debra in the fall. Consequently, after explaining Debra's situation, Nancy was able to convince the relevant district personnel working

EXHIBIT 8.2.
Appealing an Eligibility Denial

In appealing a denial of eligibility for services from government or private agencies, be knowledgeable about the eligibility criteria and use reputable evaluations to show your client, in fact, meets the criteria.

that summer to hold an individualized education meeting (IEP) prior to the fall term beginning. At the IEP meeting, the school district agreed to make a referral to the county special education program, since the district personnel in attendance concluded they did not have an appropriate program for Debra within their district. The county program had classes for children with serious emotional and behavioral problems. No assessment of Debra by the district occurred that summer, however, because there was no one there even to review Debra's case.

What Had Gone Wrong?

Debra had been placed in a new foster home in the summer. Many school districts run extended year programs in the summer for children with disabilities. This district, however, because of its small size, did not have programs at all, even during the regular school year, for children with serious emotional and behavioral problems. The district had an arrangement whereby it would refer students with serious emotional disturbances to the county schools program. Furthermore, the district had few special education and assessment staff members working in the summer, making it almost impossible to get anything done during that time of the school year.

Advocacy Considerations

State law was clear that school districts did not have to initiate the special education assessment process or hold IEP meetings for children whose cases were referred to them in the summer (Special Education Programs, 2005). Days between school terms and semesters were excluded from the state assessment timelines. The problem with the state law, in relation to CPS placing foster youth with disabilities in homes during the summer months, was that some, like Debra, were likely to be out of school for a long period of time. The district in which Lucille's foster home was located had few special education and assessment personnel working in the summer months and, furthermore, did not have an appropriate school program to meet Debra's needs. A referral to the county schools program, which the school recommended for Debra, required an IEP meeting and a subsequent referral to the county. Nancy, through her advocacy skills, was able to get the school district personnel who were working in the summer to hold an IEP meeting and start the referral process to the county program. Once the referral was made, the county program then took thirty to sixty days to hold an IEP meeting and finalize the school placement. A foster child in Debra's situation would be out of school until the county held its own IEP meeting and a county school placement was written on the child's IEP. Since Nancy had gotten the district to hold the IEP meeting in the summer, theoretically it should have shortened somewhat the amount of time Debra would be out of school (see Exhibit 8.3).

Psychiatric Inpatient Hospitalization

As the summer progressed, Debra's behavior began to deteriorate. Nancy spoke with Lucille toward the end of August and was informed that Debra's behavior had been out of control for the past two weeks. Lucille told her that Debra would scream and yell and run around the house as if she was wound up. She had been talking incessantly about having sex, making comments such as "pump it to me hard," which she then would deny having said and claimed another girl in the home was the one who had made the comment. Even though Lucille specifically had hired someone to help her with Debra, she relayed how difficult she still was to care for. What made it particularly stressful was that Debra was at home all the time, since she was not in school. Lucille began to worry that Debra needed a different residential setting, one that would provide more structure for her and help control her behavior.

Lucille continued to care for Debra in her home through September. Debra still was not attending school. By the beginning of October,

---

EXHIBIT 8.3.
Change of Placement in the Summer

If a child who receives special education services requires a school program during the summer months, prior to a home placement change occurring check with the new school district to determine if it will quickly be able to put the child in an appropriate program once the change of placement occurs.

Debra was displaying physical aggression toward adults and the other youths in the foster home. She had run away from the home on several occasions. She also appeared to be hallucinating. With the help of Debra's social worker, Lucille had Debra admitted to a children's unit of a local psychiatric hospital. Because Debra was evaluated as being a danger to herself and to others by the hospital psychiatric staff, she was admitted on a compulsory seventy-two-hour hold (LPS Act, 1968). The psychiatric staff had witnessed her physical aggression. Also, Debra admitted to them she was having auditory and visual hallucinations and suicidal thoughts.

The recommendation from the psychiatric staff was that Debra was in need of intensive psychiatric treatment in a structured inpatient setting for three to six months. The director of children's inpatient services at the hospital wrote a letter to the judge of the juvenile court requesting that an order be issued for inpatient treatment, including medication and behavioral psychotherapeutic interventions.

By this time, Debra's behavior no longer made her eligible for involuntary hospital placement since she no longer was considered by the psychiatric team to be a danger to herself and others. Nevertheless, she told her social worker that she would agree to remain hospitalized voluntarily.

A court hearing was required, however, to determine whether Debra would remain in the psychiatric hospital. At this point, Debra had to agree before the judge to remain hospitalized since it would be a voluntary placement. The hearing was scheduled. At the hearing, when the judge asked Debra whether she agreed to remain in the hospital voluntarily, although she just had told her social worker that she would, she informed the judge that she did not want to remain hospitalized. Consequently, the judge ordered her to be discharged from the hospital by midnight that very night.

Foster Home Closes Down

Since no one had anticipated Debra's immediate release from the hospital, plans had not been made to return her to Lucille's home. Once Debra's social worker realized that she had to find Debra an immediate place to live, she made a frantic call to Lucille, who readily came and picked up Debra from the courthouse and took her back to her home.

It was now the end of October and there still was no school placement for Debra. An IEP meeting was held in the first week of November and a county-run program called Apollo, which she previously had attended, was recommended for her. However, when Lucille saw the program, she realized that it was not an appropriate setting for Debra because there were busy streets with quite a lot of traffic surrounding the school and the campus was not secure. Her concern was that Debra would run out into the streets, if given the opportunity, with no thought of the oncoming traffic. Consequently, the county decided instead it would recommend a nonpublic school placement for Debra, but the board of education would have to approve it first at an upcoming meeting that was scheduled a couple of weeks away. In the meantime, a teacher from the school district was to start working with Debra at the foster home.

Lucille made an appointment at a nonpublic school that had been recommended for Debra. She visited the school and, along with Debra, had an interview with the staff. However, before Debra started attending, Lucille's foster home was shut down without warning due to a problem with her state foster care license. Consequently, Debra was removed from her home and again placed at the emergency shelter. At the shelter, she immediately started attending the on-grounds school run by the county education agency.

What Had Gone Wrong?

It is not clear from Advocacy Services records on Debra the specific problem with Lucille's foster care license that led her foster home to be shut down so abruptly. The social worker clearly still had faith in this foster mother since, even with her foster home closed, he still considered having her become Debra's legal guardian.

Independent of the licensing problem, a serious ongoing problem with Debra's placement at Lucille's was that, for all the months she was with this foster mother, Debra never had been enrolled in a school. Lucille did her best and Nancy provided some important advocacy in the beginning, but the way in which the referral process between the school district and the county schools worked resulted in Debra not having a school placement for five months.

Another Foster Home and School Placement

Within a month of Debra's return to the emergency shelter, she was placed in another foster home where Shirley was the foster parent. This time, Debra immediately was enrolled in school and placed in a public special education program for students with severe cognitive disabilities.

At the IEP meeting, the decision of the team was that Debra would remain in her current classroom only as an interim thirty-day placement. The team members felt that Debra would benefit from association with classmates nearer to her language abilities. Consequently, her CPS social worker would investigate a county school program that the district was recommending to see if it was an appropriate school setting for Debra. The team also decided that Debra would not go with her classmates on community outings because of her suicidal tendencies that had been exhibited on a previous outing.

Debra's school placement never was changed to the county program. Debra was removed from Shirley's foster home before a school placement change was able to occur. Shirley became increasingly concerned about Debra's safety in her home. On three separate occasions, Debra had run out into the street and laid down screaming that she wanted to die. Her social worker decided to return Debra to the emergency shelter for her own safety.

What Had Gone Wrong?

The structure, support, and expertise needed to care appropriately for Debra were not available in the foster home in which CPS had placed her.

Return to the Emergency Shelter

Prevention/Intervention

Once Debra returned to the emergency shelter, a behavioral assistant was assigned to her full time because she was considered a danger to herself. The social worker, being particularly concerned about Debra's dangerous behaviors, initiated an assessment by a psychologist to gain insight into her needs and the type of placement she required. The social worker felt that Debra should not be placed in another nonsecure foster home.

The psychologist's evaluation indicated that Debra's thinking was extremely concrete and simplistic and that she had little ability to engage in planning or thinking ahead. She could complete simple tasks but was stymied when they became more difficult. The report concluded that Debra's lowered cognitive functioning was attributable to her mild mental retardation rather than the result of her mental illness or deprivation in her early years.

Debra's case again was turned over to the Special Placement Unit of the emergency shelter. The staff in this unit wanted the Regional Center to be involved in securing a new placement for Debra, but a decision about her eligibility had never been received.

Advocacy Considerations

The reason that Regional Center eligibility was important for Debra was because it had both immediate and long-term consequences. Of present concern was locating an appropriate placement for her. The Regional Center was more knowledgeable than CPS about placement options in the community that were appropriate for individuals with developmental disabilities. Furthermore, if Debra were eligible for Regional Center services then that agency, along with CPS, would share the cost of her placement. Once Debra turned eighteen (or nineteen under certain circumstances) and was no longer eligible for services from CPS, the Regional Center then would be the agency responsible for her housing and other needs.

Regional Center Denial

A call was made to the Regional Center to ascertain why a decision that should have arrived within five days took ten months. After the call, the Regional Center letter finally arrived and stated that Debra had been denied eligibility. The multidisciplinary team that reviewed Debra's case determined that she did not have a "substantial handicapping condition similar to mental retardation or requiring similar services," which was required under state law (Lanterman Developmental Disabilities Services Act [Lanterman Act], 1968).

Nancy requested a state-level hearing to contest the Regional Center's denial of services to Debra. The hearing, however, never took place. In the interim, the Regional Center sent a psychologist to the emergency shelter to evaluate Debra, the same psychologist who previously had evaluated her, and this time he found her eligible for services. The day before the hearing was scheduled to begin Nancy received a call from the Regional Center's attorney informing her that Debra in fact had been found eligible. Nancy immediately called the hearing officer assigned to the case to let him know that there had been a settlement and there was no need for the hearing to proceed.

The letter that followed, confirming Debra's eligibility, stated, "It was determined that [Debra] does have a substantially handicapping condition and that she requires services similar to those services that are provided to mentally retarded persons . . . therefore [Debra] has been determined eligible for Regional Center services." Once Nancy received the letter confirming Debra's Regional Center eligibility, she formally dismissed the state hearing.

Advocacy Considerations

Why did the Regional Center finally grant Debra the eligibility for services when twice previously it had turned her down? The answer undoubtedly lies in the fact that Nancy was willing to take the case to a state-level hearing. Equally important, however, was the recent evaluation confirming Debra's mental retardation independent of her mental illness. Furthermore, there were professionals who had worked closely with Debra at the emergency shelter—specifically, the psychiatrist, the school psychologist, and the speech and language specialist—who were willing to testify at the hearing that Debra had mental retardation.

The irony was that the psychologist who originally had evaluated Debra and found that she did not qualify for services was now the same psychologist who certified her need for the same types of services that are required for individuals with mental retardation. This psychologist's confirmation of her need for the same types of services as those with mental retardation is what enabled the Regional Center to find her eligible for services.

Placement in a Residential Treatment Facility

After Nancy had filed for a hearing with the Regional Center, but before it was known that the Regional Center had granted Debra eligibility, CPS had sent a packet of information about Debra to a residential treatment facility in a nearby county. This residential facility, Cavanaugh, was the same one Robert had been in for a short period of time. It catered to residents who had developmental disabilities (specifically those with mental retardation). Cavanaugh accepted Debra and she began her placement there right around her fourteenth birthday. Those involved in her case hoped that Cavanaugh would turn out to be a long-term placement for her, although there were some concerns about whether the facility would be equipped to deal adequately with her behavior.

In order to monitor how the placement at Cavanaugh was working for Debra, Nancy kept in close contact with her counselor at the facility. Initially, Debra did fairly well there. But gradually Nancy started hearing reports about Debra's resistant, and sometimes aggressive, behavior, particularly in relation to the afternoon and early evening childcare staff on the residential unit. Nancy decided to go to Cavanaugh to meet with the staff members, hoping to forge a relationship with them and together try to figure out what brought on Debra's behavior problems in the afternoon. Nancy also hoped to encourage the staff to maintain Debra's placement at this facility, even if the behavior problems persisted.

But, ultimately, Nancy was unsuccessful. Debra assaulted the afternoon staff one too many times. In what turned out to be the last two weeks of her stay at Cavanaugh, Debra was admitted to a psychiatric hospital twice for her aggressive behavior and then promptly was discharged from Cavanaugh. As it turned out, Debra's placement at Cavanaugh lasted only for a little over three months.

What Had Gone Wrong?

While Cavanaugh's treatment focus was on individuals with developmental disabilities, it was a facility, as was apparent in Robert's case, which was not prepared to deal with residents with significant behavior problems.

A Group Home for Individuals with Development Disabilities

Debra once again entered the emergency shelter. This time she stayed there for six months before being placed in the Gardner Home, a six-bed group home for individuals with developmental disabilities. Once placed in this group home, Debra immediately started attending Markham High, a public special education school for students with moderate to severe developmental delays. Pam, staff attorney at Advocacy Services, had started working on the case with Nancy, so she and I decided to go and observe the school program and visit a bit with Debra.

At the school, we talked with the principal who indicated that Debra seemed properly placed there, even though her verbal skills were better than most of the other students. It turned out we were unable to observe Debra in class because our discussion with the principal took us into the lunch hour, but we did get time to visit with Debra. She was a delight to talk to, a real storyteller with a good sense of humor.

Debra did eventually start to have some problems in school, but they did not involve engaging in challenging or threatening behavior. What she did instead was to tell the teacher she was not feeling well in order to be sent to the nurse's office, which then removed her from class and doing work that she did not want to do. The teacher and others in the school finally realized what Debra was doing and quickly put a stop to it.

How to Pay for Debra's Placement at the Group Home

Since this group home exclusively was for individuals with development disabilities, the cost of housing residents there always had been paid for by the Regional Center. The Regional Center had developed its own specific payment contracts with the homes with which it contracted.

The first problem that arose in regard to this group home placement for Debra was that CPS did not have a contract with the Gardner Group Home and, consequently, could not figure out how to pay for Debra's placement there. Because of this payment problem, Debra was in jeopardy of being terminated from the Gardner Group Home. From Nancy's perspective, this would have been disastrous since it was so difficult to find a placement for Debra and she seemed to be doing well in this one. In order to prevent Debra's termination from this group home, Nancy spent considerable time helping CPS to work out how to pay for the group home. The way it finally was worked out was that CPS would send the money for Debra's placement at the Gardner Home to the Regional Center and the Regional Center then, through its contract with the Gardner Group Home, would forward the funding for Debra to the home.

Advocacy Considerations

Although most of Nancy's dealings with CPS over issues related to Debra had been with her caseworker, she realized that she would not be able to solve the payment problem simply by continuing to talk with this worker. Nancy decided to go up the chain of command at CPS. She contacted the senior administrative staff at the agency to discuss how CPS could pay for the Gardner Group Home and to convince them of the importance of Debra remaining in this particular group home. Ultimately, it took the involvement of the director of CPS to truly work out the process for paying for Debra's placement. The bureaucratic nature and insularity of CPS made it such that no one below the director had the authority to work out a creative solution to funding an interagency placement (see Exhibit 8.4).

Behavior Problems Jeopardize Group Home Placement

Not surprisingly, the next problem that arose concerned Debra's sometimes erratic, and frequently challenging, behavior. The primary

---

EXHIBIT 8.4.
Follow the Chain of Command

If a bureaucratic problem arises that jeopardizes an appropriate foster or group home placement for a hard to place child, go up the chain of command in the placing agency until you get to the administrative level where the problem can be addressed.

caretaker at the Gardner Group Home had serious concerns about Debra's lack of cooperation, threatening behavior, and combativeness. This conduct made it quite probable that Debra would quickly be terminated from the home.

Pam paid a visit to the caretaker in charge of the group home to get a better sense of how things were going. The caretaker complained to Pam that they had not been told the truth about Debra's range of challenging behaviors when determining whether to accept her. The only behavior they had been informed about, she said, was that periodically Debra engaged in dangerous activities (e.g., lying down in the middle of the street) when she became suicidal. The caretaker said she was prepared to deal with the suicidal behavior but had not anticipated that Debra would be extremely challenging on an ongoing basis.

A week after the meeting with the caretaker, Pam called the group home to follow up on how Debra was faring there. During this conversation, the caretaker expressed serious concern about Debra's refusal to cooperate in doing her after-school household chores. The caretaker described these chores as part of their program for teaching independent living skills and that Debra required constant counseling during the time these chores were to be completed in order to get her to begin them as well as keep her functioning and to remain on task. The caretaker indicated that she wanted the Regional Center to provide counseling to Debra to help with her behavior but had been unable to make contact with the requisite Regional Center caseworker.

Hoping to maintain Debra in the Gardner Group Home, Pam knew that the caretaker desperately needed some additional help and that Debra's difficult behaviors very quickly had to be diminished. The caretaker gave Pam the name of a psychologist who worked for the Regional Center and who she wanted to work with Debra. However, the caretaker had been unsuccessful in her attempts to arrange for services from this psychologist through the Regional Center.

Intervention

After Pam's conversation with the caretaker, she immediately called and left a message for the psychologist. He promptly returned Pam's call and after her vivid description of the behavior problems that the caretaker was having with Debra and how this behavior was jeopardizing the placement, the psychologist agreed to meet with Debra and the caretaker to develop a behavioral program, since Debra was a client of the Regional Center. Within the week, the psychologist had a meeting with Debra and the caretaker and had developed a behavior management plan for the staff in the group home to use in working with her. While the caretaker had a "wait and see" attitude as to whether Debra could successfully be managed in the group home, the psychologist was hopeful that Debra's difficult behaviors could be reduced rather quickly.

The behavior management system the psychologist set up was a positive behavioral incentive program. The goals of the program specifically were to reduce Debra's tantrums and increase her compliant behavior. Debra selected the major incentives that she wanted to work toward, like attending a school dance or having a special celebration for her birthday. She also received smaller incentives on a daily basis to keep her motivated. The psychologist called Pam about a week later to report that the behavioral program was working and Debra's behavior was improving.

What Had Gone Wrong?

Why was the caretaker at the Gardner Group Home unable to arrange for a psychologist to develop a behavioral management plan for Debra? The Regional Center, because of budget cuts, was understaffed and, at that point, Debra did not have an assigned caseworker. Consequently, the caretaker was unable to arrange for the behavioral services that Debra needed in order to stay in the group home.

Advocacy Considerations

Pam contacted the psychologist directly whom the caretaker had suggested. This psychologist had been providing services to clients of the Regional Center for some time and, therefore, was able to negotiate the Regional Center system and initiate services for Debra even though she had no caseworker to authorize these services. Pam had provided the psychologist with enough details about Debra's history, and particularly her history of behavior problems leading to failed placements, so he felt he had sufficient background information to begin his work.

The Need for a Saturday Program

Pam continued to check in with the caretaker on a weekly basis about Debra's behavior and to try to support the caretaker in her work with Debra. This continued contact and support by Pam was particularly important because there still was no CPS caseworker assigned to Debra's case.

Debra's behavior generally was improved, particularly during the school week. However, there still were times when she became difficult to deal with and sometimes frightened the other children in the home by her threatening behavior. Pam's constant contact with the caretaker seems to have paid off, however, because even when Debra's behavior was challenging the caretaker continued to maintain Debra in the placement.

One day the caretaker called Pam to let her know that the behavior problems Debra was having on the weekends had become so constant that weekend childcare workers felt they no longer could deal with her. The caretaker indicated that something had to be done soon or Debra would no longer be able to remain in the placement.

Pam immediately contacted the psychologist who had worked out the behavior program for Debra and requested his involvement again. He went out to observe the situation and ultimately helped identify some incentives that he thought would motivate Debra to improve her behavior on the weekends. However, the psychologist reported to Pam that the weekend childcare workers were not really implementing the behavior management program that he had set up for Debra in the first place. He thought the staff needed ongoing help to ensure that the behavior management program was being implemented and implemented properly. Consequently, Pam requested that the Regional Center fund someone to come into the group home on a regular basis to ensure that the behavior management program was being properly implemented.

Since Debra did not have a Regional Center case manager, Pam was referred to the case manager director. After several conversations, she informed Pam that, because of limited funding, the Regional Center could only fund someone to come into the group home twice over a two-month period.

Knowing that the weekend problem with Debra had not really been solved, Pam requested that the Regional Center provide respite services for the group home staff by paying for a Saturday program for Debra to attend. Pam could not get the case manager director to identify an appropriate Saturday program or expedite the respite services request. Finally, Pam wrote a letter to both the executive director and the case management director of the Regional Center stating that Debra's individual program plan at the agency did not meet her needs because it did not include respite care or a Saturday program. The letter went on to say that if there could not be agreement on respite services for Debra, then Advocacy Services would have to appeal this issue. Pam also engaged in a search to locate an appropriate Saturday respite program for Debra, which she did locate. After receiving Pam's letter, the Regional Center finally agreed to fund the Saturday program that Pam had identified, which ultimately relieved much of the stress in the group home related to Debra's behavior and allowed Debra to remain in this placement.

What Had Gone Wrong?

Although the Regional Center funded a psychologist to develop a behavior management plan to address Debra's behavior problems (i.e., tantrums and noncompliance), there had been no services put in place to ensure the behavior plan was being properly implemented. Furthermore, in developing Debra's individual program plan, there had been no consideration as to the need for respite services for those who cared for Debra at the group home. Given the fact that it was difficult to keep Debra in a placement for any length of time, it is hard to imagine why a comprehensive program was not put together to address all of Debra's needs and the needs of those who cared for her. The Regional Center had undergone some budget cuts and, consequently, was not readily providing the full range of services necessary to address their clients' needs.

Advocacy Considerations

Pam engaged in several activities to try to maintain Debra is her group home placement. First, she maintained weekly contact with the group home caretaker. Because of this contact, the caretaker did not request that Debra be removed from her home even when she contin-ued to be difficult to handle. Instead, the caretaker contacted Pam and together they tried to solve the difficult problem of Debra's behavior and provide respite for the staff.

Second, Pam requested needed services for Debra from the Re-gional Center. When the Regional Center did not provide the services that were requested, Pam wrote a letter letting the executive director of the Regional Center know that she would appeal a denial of the ser-vices. She also let the executive director know that she would prefer to negotiate an agreement rather than have to follow through on an appeal.

Third, Pam located an appropriate Saturday program herself for Debra when no one at the Regional Center followed through on search-ing for a program. Consequently, there was an actual, known program that Pam was requesting, which ultimately made it more difficult to deny (see Exhibit 8.5).

The Law Changes Creating a Problem in Funding the Group Home

What happened next was unforeseen. The state law changed, mak-ing it no longer possible for CPS to fund placements in for-profit (as opposed to nonprofit) facilities. The Gardner Group Home, it turned out, was a for-profit facility.

By this time, a CPS social worker had been assigned to Debra's case. During one of Pam's conversations with the social worker, she informed Pam that Debra would have to be moved from the Gardner

---

EXHIBIT 8.5.
Supporting a Caregiver

A good strategy to use to keep a difficult-to-place child in a place-ment is to support the caregiver. This can be done by: (1) calling on a regular basis to see how the caregiver is faring with the child, (2) re-quest support for the caregiver when problems arise, and (3) use appropriate advocacy strategies when relevant agencies are not forth-coming with needed support.

Group Home because CPS no longer could pay for the placement in light of the new state law. Not wanting Debra to be moved from this placement because she had been more stable there than anywhere else, Pam immediately went into action. She called the CPS special placement and contracts units to try to work out continued payment to the group home for Debra. When she was not successful with these two units of CPS, she proceeded to contact senior administrative staff at CPS. Her conversations with these staff were not fruitful in ensuring CPS would be able to continue paying for Debra's for-profit group home. Finally, Pam went into court and requested from the judge that Debra not be removed from her current group home without a court hearing. The judge granted this court order. Consequently, Debra remained in the Gardner Group Home; and, notwithstanding the new state law, CPS continued to pay for Debra's placement there.

Advocacy Considerations

When CPS senior administrators believed they no longer could pay for the group home in which Debra was placed because of a new state law disallowing payment for placements in for-profit facilities, Pam ultimately sought (and was granted) an order from the juvenile court to prevent Debra's removal from the group home without a court hearing. This strategy allowed CPS to continue to pay for the for-profit facility by referencing the court order. The court order was seen and accepted by CPS administrators and contract officers as overriding the provisions of a new state law.

CONCLUSION

Debra was a challenge to keep in a home placement and to get her finally enrolled in school. She sorely had tried the patience and skills of devoted and well-respected foster parents. A residential treatment facility for individuals with developmental disabilities could not handle her difficult behavior. Debra's dual diagnosis—mental retardation and a psychiatric disorder—made her difficult to maintain in any placement.

CPS had to work with the Regional Center and private agencies designated by the state to provide or procure services for individuals with developmental disabilities to locate a group home for Debra. The Regional Center identified such a group home, which housed individuals with mental retardation, and Debra was placed there. A public school program that met her needs was located nearby.

The group home placement, however, was jeopardized. With the advent of a change in state law, problems arose related to CPS funding this group home placement. Problems also occurred because the group home needed more support in order to maintain Debra in this placement. Strong, consistent advocacy efforts on behalf of Debra were necessary to bring about solutions to both of these problems. These solutions eventually brought about needed placement stability for Debra.

SUMMARY

The purpose of this chapter was to show why child protective services must be cognizant of the special education services a school district has prior to placing a foster child in a home in a particular school district. The chapter also shows that timing of the placement also can affect the immediate enrollment of a foster child in a school or whether the child may be out of school for many months. In addition, this chapter highlights how thinking "outside the box" may be at times be necessary in order to fund certain group home placements and also supplement their services to provide placement stability for difficult-to-place youth with special needs.

Chapter 9

Patty: Funding a Unique Program

INTRODUCTION

The case of Patty addresses the troubling issue of what happens to a foster child when a placement best suited to her specific needs is available but unaffordable. Patty is another child whose permanency, treatment, and educational needs had not been addressed by the numerous foster and group home placements in which she had been placed without success. Each failed placement occurred because the caregivers did not have the tools to affect her difficult and frequently dangerous behaviors. Most settings in which she had been placed assumed she had the ability to conform her behavior to the caregiver's demands if she so chose. This assumption was far from the case.

Patty had required neurosurgery to repair a fractured skull and was left cognitively impaired from brain damage. The injury was a result of a car accident when she was three. The driver of the car was her father. She also was a victim of sexual abuse after the accident, allegedly by family members. She entered the foster care system when she was ten, but CPS did not appear to take into account her traumatic brain injury in locating proper home and school placements for her.

Patty required a treatment setting where there was expertise in working with those who had traumatic brain injuries. She also was badly in need of professionals working with her to help her understand not only the problems she had related to the sexual abuse, but also later the death of her father as well as her history of out-of-home placement.

Unlike some of the other children described in this book, a treatment setting that seemed perfect for Patty was identified finally.

doi:10.1300/5136_09

It consisted of a residential program where an interdisciplinary team of brain injury specialists would address Patty's severe maladaptive behavior and increase her independence by helping her gain skills and develop strategies to compensate for her brain injury. The problem, however, was how to pay for this facility, since the cost was substantially more than the rate that CPS paid for residential treatment programs for foster youth. This chapter details the various avenues that were pursued and the advocacy strategies that were used trying to piece together interagency funding so that Patty finally could get the treatment she needed.

CASE STUDY OF PATTY

Early Years

Patty's parents, Marsha and John, divorced when she was an infant. Marsha subsequently committed suicide when Patty was two by overdosing on drugs. At three, an automobile accident occurred that left Patty with serious brain damage. John, her father, was the driver of the vehicle and was presumed to have been driving under the influence of alcohol. Patty had been thrown from the car during the head-on collision, which severely injured her father's back and legs, requiring numerous surgeries and leaving him permanently disabled.

Patty was in a coma for three months. When she came out of it, her functioning was at the level of a three- or four-month old child. She had to relearn all the skills she already had mastered, but no longer remembered how to do, such as walking, talking, and using the toilet. She also had no memory of who her father was. Although she eventually regained most of her skills, her functioning now was in the range of mild mental retardation and she had pervasive developmental delays. Specific areas of difficulty identified at this time were in certain language and memory functions. As a result of Patty's brain damage and cognitive delays, she became eligible for services from the Regional Center when she was three and a half (see Exhibit 9.1).

The Regional Center funded her attendance at a special preschool program to enhance her development and, as a result, she was able to start elementary school in a regular kindergarten class. However, when she was in the first grade, she was evaluated and became eligible for

EXHIBIT 9.1.
Placement History

Age	Placement	Maltreatment	School
10 yrs. 4 mos.	Foster Home	Abuse	N/A
10 yrs. 5 mos.	Father	N/A	
12 yrs. 2 mos.	Johnson Group Home	Neglect	Grover Jr. High
13-15 yrs.	Foster Home		N/A
	Gramercy Group Home		
	Foster Home		
	Donaldson Group Home		
	Westcomb Group Home		
	Samuels Group Home		
	Beverly Group Home		
	Waterton Group Home		
15 yrs. 2 mos.	Foster Home		N/A
15 yrs. 9 mos.	Foster Home		N/A
15 yrs. 9 mos.	Foster Home		N/A
15 yrs. 10 mos.	Foster Home		N/A
	Emergency Shelter		Shelter School
16 yrs.	Cavanaugh Residential		Cavanaugh School
16 yrs. 3 mos.	Psychiatric Hospital		Hospital School
16 yrs. 4 mos.	Emergency Shelter		Shelter School
17 yrs. 6 mos.	Rehab Residential		On-site teacher

N/A = No records available.

Jr. High = Junior High or Middle School.

special education services and was placed in a full-day special education class. She remained in special education classes throughout her school history.

When Patty was seven, her father remarried. She lived with him and Sally, her new stepmother, and three stepbrothers, Jason, Rick, and Roger. Life appeared fairly stable for Patty at this time, with Sally taking an active interest in her and her education. However, Sally and John's marriage lasted only for three years. They separated when Patty was ten.

Sexual Abuse

Shortly after Patty's father and stepmother separated, Patty revealed that Jason, her older stepbrother, had molested her. Her father contacted CPS to report the sexual molestation. During the course of the investigation, Patty claimed that her father also had sexually molested her, when she was a small child.

Prevention

Patty was removed from her father's home by CPS and placed in a foster home with foster parents Ed and Marie. During her stay there, Marie reported to CPS that Patty had engaged in sexual activities with a seven-year-old foster child who also lived in the home.

Sexual Abuse Not Substantiated

Since the allegations of sexual abuse by her father were not substantiated, Patty was returned to John's home. Without substantiated abuse or neglect by her father, CPS could not continue to keep Patty in out-of-home placement.

Request for Voluntary Removal

Several months later, however, CPS received a report from Lisa and George, a family that had provided childcare to Patty intermittently. They reported that, while staying overnight with them, Patty had gotten up at about 3:00 a.m. and climbed on an adult male in the home and began rubbing against him sexually. They claimed she had done the same thing to a three-year-old in their home on another occasion. Consequently, CPS suggested to Patty's father that they place her in a residential facility, in an attempt to correct her inappropriate sexual behavior. Patty's father, however, refused to have her placed in the facility, but, because he was about to be hospitalized for needed surgery, he arranged to have her stay with an aunt and uncle.

Patty remained with her aunt and uncle until she told school district personnel that her uncle had molested her. Although she quickly denied the accusation, claiming that it was only a dream, her aunt and uncle felt they no longer could care for her.

CPS Files a Petition

CPS filed a petition with the juvenile court alleging that Patty's father had neglected her in that he failed to adequately supervise her and to cooperate in obtaining necessary counseling and treatment to correct her inappropriate sexual behavior.

Prevention/Intervention

Patty, a little over twelve now, was taken from her father's home and placed in a group home facility where she was to receive assessment and treatment of her emotional and behavioral problems.

Group Home Placement

Intervention

The Johnson Group Home, where CPS placed Patty, was for emotionally disturbed girls, ages ten to seventeen. She also attended a public school program for behaviorally disordered students at Grover Middle School. Virginia, the owner of the group home, and other childcare staff at the group home described Patty's behavior, at this time, as exposing herself to others, using explicit sexual talk with male peers, and engaging in excessive touching of peers and staff. As a consequence of her inappropriate behaviors, the group home staff prohibited her access to community outings, confiscated her personal possessions (such as her radio, games, posters for the wall, and make-up), and restricted her to her bedroom for time-outs.

Patty's Regional Center caseworker had serious concerns as to whether the Johnson Group Home program was appropriate for Patty. Consequently, the caseworker sent a behavior specialist to evaluate the program's effectiveness.

The behavior specialist noted in his report that Patty had been deprived of all her possessions, was having an almost impossible time earning them back, and, in addition, was being prohibited from going on outings. The specialist emphasized not only was she unable to articulate the house rules, she also was unable to explain how one earned back possessions and outings.

What Had Gone Wrong?

The behavior specialist delineated why the Johnson Group Home did not have an effective treatment program. He reported that there were no individualized behavior plans for the girls who resided there and there did not appear to be much consistency in the programming. The conclusion of the behavior specialist was that the program was inappropriate for Patty as well as any other Regional Center client.

Foster Care Drift

What followed for Patty was placement by CPS in a series of foster and group homes, none of which worked out. Her typical behavior at these homes was running away and presumably seeking out relationships with men.

By the time Patty was fifteen, she had been in eight different foster or group homes and her academic functioning was at a beginning elementary school level. She only could read very simple words, such as *cat* and *run,* and she was just learning to tell time and do basic money skills. She had to be supervised at all times, since if left alone she would get in cars with total strangers. She was described in psychological reports at this time as insecure and moody, and could become rageful and hostile when she did not get her way. She spoke and acted like a seven-year-old, but, at times, behaved as if she were three.

At this point, she was placed in the home of Molly and Sam, a couple who had lived near her when she was young. Although Molly and Sam seemed committed to her, at least at first, and were interested in becoming her legal guardians, after seven months they decided they could no longer care for her. Patty was having a particularly hard time because her father had recently died. She intentionally burned herself while being taught to use an iron. She ran away from her foster parents' home on several occasions, claiming to have been raped while she was gone. Emergency room evaluations proved that it was not the case. Finally, she alleged that Sam had sexually molested her.

What followed was placement in three different foster homes (i.e., with the Darby's, the Thomas', and then the Ross') in three weeks, running away from all of them. Then, for a period of time, she was living on the streets, allegedly exchanging sexual favors for housing and drugs.

When Patty returned to the Ross' foster home, she was detained by CPS and placed at the county emergency shelter. An evaluation done while she was in the shelter, diagnosed her with mild mental retardation and organic brain syndrome (a term referring to physical disorders, such as trauma-induced head injuries, that cause decreased mental function). Also noted in this report was that she became overwhelmed by thoughts and fantasies that were poorly organized, and that she had limited internal resources with which to cope with stressful situations.

Two months later, she was placed at a residential treatment facility for youngsters with developmental delays, called Cavanaugh Residential, the same facility in which Richard and Debra had been placed for a short time. She lasted there for three months, before running away and being picked up by the police. The residential facility then had her hospitalized in an adolescent psychiatric unit because she claimed to be hearing voices telling her to run away from the facility and to kill herself. She remained in the hospital for three months, the hospital psychiatric team having concluded she would not be safe outside a locked environment. She attended the hospital school and received some individual and group psychological therapy, when she was stable enough to participate. The psychiatrist worked to reduce her hallucinations and self-destructive behaviors with medication. Upon discharge, CPS had not located another placement for her, so she was returned to the emergency shelter.

Advocacy Services Appointed as Co-Counsel

Two months after Patty returned to the emergency shelter, Nancy was appointed as one of her attorneys by the juvenile court. The other attorney, Rachael Woodman, had already been working on the case and had located a residential facility, called Rehab Residential Center, whose program was specially designed to rehabilitate those who had received head injuries.

Shortly after Nancy was appointed to represent Patty, she and I discussed her case and decided we would try to push each of the agencies that had some responsibility for Patty's placement in the hope that we ultimately might succeed in having her placed in Rehab Residential Center. We started with the Regional Center.

The Regional Center

We asked the Regional Center to determine if there were any programs in the state, other than Rehab Residential Center, that would be appropriate for Patty. After conducting a statewide search of facilities with which the agency contracted, the Regional Center's placement coordinator concluded that there were no appropriate community placements for her anywhere in the state. Nancy then requested that the Regional Center provide funding for Rehab Residential Center for Patty.

Rather than authorize funding for the head trauma program, the Regional Center instead expressed concern, along with CPS, as to whether Patty would be able to benefit from the program, since the accident causing her head trauma had occurred quite some time ago. In fact, in a case staffing report, the clinical staff explicitly denied that the training and treatment Patty would receive from Rehab Residential Center would be of any benefit to her. They argued instead that she would need long-term care, perhaps years, in a stable environment that would prevent her from endangering herself. This was the Regional Center's way of saying she belonged in the state hospital.

What Had Gone Wrong?

The Regional Center did not want to fund Patty's placement at Rehab Residential Center, since it was significantly more costly than any other group home, residential, or state hospital option. Since the Regional Center's state search of group home or residential placement facilities for Patty had determined there were none that were appropriate, the Regional Center and CPS argued that Patty should be placed in the state hospital. Regional Center and CPS staff may well have believed that Patty would not benefit from Rehab Residential Center, since her traumatic brain injury occurred when she was three; but there was no doubt that cost considerations played a major role in their decision.

A Court-Ordered Evaluation

In trying to determine whether Patty's needs in fact would adequately be met in a six to nine month stay at Rehab Residential Center, Nancy requested that the juvenile court order a neuropsychological examination of Patty. The judge granted the order.

The neuropsychologist who evaluated Patty found significantly lowered intellectual and adaptive functioning resulting from her head trauma, which led to poor academic learning. His opinion was that anxiety and other clinical conditions did not appear to be primary, although depression and anxiety did have some impact on her ability to perform. His testing of Patty clearly pointed to right hemisphere brain damage. She had visual-spatial difficulties, along with memory impairment that was described as general in nature, rather than specific to verbal or nonverbal material. While her fund of knowledge was very poor, her learning curve suggested the ability to learn, but at a slower rate than others her age. She also had difficulty shifting from one situation to another, especially in new situations. Her judgment and impulse control were impaired. She tended to take a concrete attitude toward most tasks and had a poor ability to engage in abstractions. Her ability to concentrate or sustain attention was poor. He found that Patty's self-esteem and sense of adequacy were poor as well. When faced with more complex tasks, she tended to give up quickly and become very frustrated. His opinion was that it was not uncommon that she had socially unacceptable behavior as part of her overall condition. However, she showed potential for learning and for more successful social relationships.

The neuropsychologist, contrary to the opinion of the Regional Center and CPS staff, recommended that Patty receive a rehabilitative approach similar to that provided to brain injured patients, despite the length of time since her head trauma. He felt this approach would provide the appropriate structure and learning models for her cognitive and behavioral difficulties. Such a program would be oriented to finding techniques suitable to her level of cognitive functioning, and she would be trained and reinforced for using compensatory aids. She also would be participating in various therapeutic and rehabilitative groups to develop her social skills, understand her cognitive difficulties, and change her unacceptable behavior.

Advocacy Considerations

Nancy knew that in order to continue pursuing funding for Rehab Residential Center for Patty, she would need a report from a professional with expertise in the area of Patty's disability. She also wanted to confirm for herself that this was the appropriate option to pursue, since professional staff at the Regional Center and CPS disagreed with this decision. Consequently, Nancy sought a court order for a neuropsychological evaluation for Patty, which was granted (see Exhibit 9.2).

Using the IEP Process

Armed with the neuropsychological evaluation, I requested an individualized education program (IEP) meeting from the school at the emergency shelter, where Patty had been placed. My purpose was to try to obtain placement for Patty in the Rehab Residential Center, based on her educational needs. It was clear that her needs, educational and otherwise, were not being met at the emergency shelter, and the only other option offered was the state hospital program, which Nancy and I deemed highly inappropriate.

In Patty's previous IEP, her eligibility for special education was on the basis of mental retardation. The only chance we had of having her placed in a residential facility because of her special educational needs

---

**EXHIBIT 9.2.
Court Orders**

Request a court order from the juvenile court for an evaluation to help determine needed components of a placement for a foster child with special needs.

was if she was classified as having an emotional disturbance under the special education laws (IDEA, 2004). This classification then would allow me to request, under state law, an evaluation by the department of mental health (DMH) to determine if Patty required residential placement to benefit educationally (Interagency Responsibilities, 2004). If DMH did determine that she required her schooling to take place in a twenty-four-hour residential program in order to be educated, DMH then would authorize the county department of social services to pay for the room and board, DMH would pay for the mental health treatment, and the local education agency (typically the child's school district) would pay for the cost of the schooling at the residential facility.

I arrived at the IEP meeting, which was held in one of the rooms at the emergency shelter school. An administrator of the school was at the meeting, as well as Patty's classroom teacher and the school psychologist. We all sat around a table in an empty classroom. I shared with the others the copies of the report by the neuropsychologist and requested that Patty's classification for special education be expanded, since mental retardation did not fully describe her disability. I suggested using a category called "multiple disabilities," which, for her, I argued, would include mental retardation, traumatic brain injury, and emotional disturbance. After some discussion, the other members of the IEP team went along with this request. I was relieved when the meeting was over; since, going into it, I was not at all sure, my request to include emotional disturbance as part of her special education eligibility description would be honored (see Exhibits 9.3, 9.4, 9.5, and 9.6).

EXHIBIT 9.3.
Multiple Disabilities

Multiple disabilities means concomitant impairments (such as mental retardation-blindness, mental retardation-orthopedic impairment, etc.), the combination of which causes such severe educational needs that they cannot be accommodated in special education programs solely for one of the impairments. The term does not include deaf-blindness. (Assistance to States, 2005)

EXHIBIT 9.4.
Traumatic Brain Injury

Traumatic brain injury means an acquired injury to the brain caused by an external physical force, resulting in total or partial functional disability or psychosocial impairment, or both, that adversely affects a child's educational performance. The term applies to open or closed head injuries resulting in impairments in one or more areas, such as cognition; language; memory; attention; reasoning; abstract thinking; judgment; problem-solving; sensory, perceptual, and motor abilities; psychosocial behavior; physical functions; information processing; and speech. The term does not apply to brain injuries that are congenital or degenerative, or to brain injuries induced by birth trauma. (Assistance to States, 2005)

EXHIBIT 9.5.
Mental Retardation

Mental retardation means significantly subaverage general intellectual functioning, existing concurrently with deficits in adaptive behavior and manifested during the developmental period that adversely affects a child's educational performance. (Assistance to States, 2004)

Sometime after the IEP meeting, I put in a call to the program head of the DMH unit who handled these special education cases. I wanted to give him some background on the case and, hopefully, convince him that Patty's case rightly warranted a residential recommendation from his department, based on the requirements of state law (see Exhibit 9.7).

Obtaining Consent for the Evaluation

The DMH program head accepted Patty's case as an appropriate referral and, consequently, decided to evaluate her need for residential placement. However, in order to do an evaluation of Patty, a signed consent form was required. Who would sign the consent form for DMH, since Patty had no parent? What was needed in this case was

EXHIBIT 9.6.
Emotional Disturbance

i. The term means a condition exhibiting one or more of the following characteristics over a long period of time and to a marked degree that adversely affects a child's educational performance:
  A. An inability to learn that cannot be explained by intellectual, sensory, or health factors.
  B. An inability to build or maintain satisfactory interpersonal relationships with peers and teachers.
  C. Inappropriate types of behavior or feelings under normal circumstances.
  D. A general pervasive mood of unhappiness or depression.
  E. A tendency to develop physical symptoms or fears associated with personal or school problems.
ii. The term includes schizophrenia. The term does not apply to children who are socially maladjusted, unless it is determined that they have an emotional disturbance. (Assistance to States, 2005, §300.8)

EXHIBIT 9.7.
Developing Relationships

Develop and nurture relationships with key players in your geographic area. These relationships may prove helpful in your advocacy efforts.

an appointed surrogate parent. But good surrogate parents are not always easy to find. We realized that Patty's previous IEPs, that were done while she was at the emergency shelter, were technically illegal, since social workers, or others who did not have the right to sign as her parent according to the law, had signed them (see Exhibit 9.8).

Nancy and I knew we had to have a proper surrogate parent appointed for Patty. The school at the emergency shelter was going to appoint a surrogate parent for her, so we decided to nominate someone we knew who we were sure would advocate for her needs. We were afraid that if the school principal at the emergency shelter

EXHIBIT 9.8.
Surrogate Parents

A surrogate parent, under special education law, is someone who is appointed by the local educational agency or the juvenile court to sign IEPs, consent to evaluations, and advocate on behalf of the child to obtain appropriate special educational services when a child has no parent, the parent cannot be located or parental rights have been limited. (IDEA, 2004)

appointed someone of his choosing it would be a person who was not savvy about special education law and would serve as a rubber stamp for the administrators of the education agency that ran the school. I breathed a sigh of relief when the principal of the emergency shelter school appointed our nomination for Patty's surrogate parent. The surrogate parent immediately signed consent for the department of mental health to evaluate Patty.

DMH Assessment Process

The department of mental health's typical procedure was to review all the school and other relevant records on a child referred to them for evaluation, talk with the child, teacher, and parents, and then write a report either recommending or denying mental health services, including residential placement. In Patty's case, since there was no parent, I gave DMH as much background information on her as I had.

After a DMH evaluator completed the evaluation of Patty, the procedure in the law was to return to another IEP meeting where a DMH representative would make a recommendation. Once the recommendation was written on the IEP, it was to be implemented immediately, according to the law (IDEA, 2004).

IEP Meeting

This IEP meeting was very well attended. It was becoming clear that a lot of people in the county were taking an interest in Patty's case because we had used the IEP process to try to obtain appropriate residential services for her. It was the first time in the county that this process had been used for this purpose with children in the emergency shelter school. The county education agency that ran this school feared that it would have to pay a portion of the residential placement costs for Patty.

There were thirteen people in attendance at the IEP meeting— representatives of all the agencies involved in her case. Those of us representing Patty were incredibly relieved when DMH approved a recommendation for residential placement for her, and also wrote this recommendation on her IEP.

The program head of DMH had written a letter to the principal of the emergency shelter school letting him know that although his agency was recommending residential placement for Patty, he anticipated great difficulty in locating a residential program that could implement her IEP (since that was what the law required). Consequently, he was going to notify the state Department of Education to rally support to help search for an appropriate program.

Approximately a month after this IEP meeting, the State Department of Education notified DMH that it was unable to identify any other appropriate residential programs for Patty in the western part of the United States. Following this notification, the DMH program head authorized Rehab Residential Center as being appropriate for Patty. In the meantime, however, the county education agency disagreed that it had any responsibility to pay for the educational portion of the residential program for Patty.

Advocacy Considerations

By recommending Rehab Residential Center for Patty, the DMH program head authorized the department of social services to pay the highest rate per month for Patty's residential care, which was only a small part of the total amount per month that was needed. Nevertheless, this was an important step.

In relation to the county education agency, the reasoning of this agency's attorney was that the county education agency was not Patty's school district of residence. Technically, this was true. Under state law, the county education agency and its school programs were not considered a school district. However, Patty did not have a school district of residence since, having no parents and no permanent residence; there was no other local educational agency responsible for her other than this county education agency.

The Regional Center Decision

Around this time, Nancy received a letter from the director of the Regional Center rejecting the request for funding for Patty's placement at Rehab Residential Center. The Regional Center not only rejected funding the program itself, but also rejected participating in funding it along with other agencies.

Nancy immediately initiated a hearing with the Regional Center to contest the denial to place Patty in Rehab Residential Center. However, the hearing officer who was to preside over the matter refused to hear the case until the educational issues were resolved. The hearing officer's reasoning here was that Patty had an IEP that recommended residential placement.

Advocacy Consideration

The Regional Center, according to state law, was not legally obligated to pay for the services for which other agencies were responsible (Lanterman Act, 1969). Consequently, the hearing officer correctly reasoned that the necessary determination of the extent to which the county education agency, any other local education agency, and DMH were responsible for Patty's placement at Rehab Residential Center had to be made before it could be determined whether the Regional Center had responsibility for any of the cost of the placement.

The Juvenile Court

Since our attempts to obtain the remainder of the funding for Rehab Residential Center for Patty were at a standstill, Nancy and her co-counsel appealed to the juvenile court to designate which agencies were responsible for paying for Patty's placement at this facility. This request led to a meeting with the judge of the juvenile court in his chambers. Nancy, I, and her co-counsel were present. The attorneys from the county education agency, the Regional Center, and CPS were also there, as well as the program head from DMH.

A new participant in the process was an attorney from the state department of education, who had flown in from the state capitol. We answered the judge's questions about the case and those who had prepared written arguments submitted them to him. The attorney for the county education agency argued, among other things, that the state department of education should be responsible for funding the placement since Patty did not have a school district of residence. The attorney representing CPS argued that since CPS stands in the place of the parents, this agency then should not bear the costs of services pursuant to an IEP, since a child's parents would not have to bear these costs under the same circumstances. This attorney argued that the responsibility to pay was either Patty's local education agency (that is, the county education agency) or the state department of education. After listening to the various oral arguments, the judge then took time to review the written arguments.

We all waited with anxious anticipation. The judge then issued a court order finding that Patty had multiple deficits as a result of a head injury—including medical, physical, cognitive, communicative, behavioral, and psychosocial. The court also found that the emergency shelter was not an appropriate placement for Patty: that she needed to be placed in a structured residential facility with an interdisciplinary team of professionals capable of addressing her problems. She required such a placement in order to achieve her potential for independent living and to benefit from an education. The judge's order clearly was written with Rehab Residential Center is mind, since no other facility fit the description.

In the court order, the county was designated as her residence and school district. Up to six months was found to be an appropriate amount of time for her to be placed at Rehab Residential Center. The court ordered that Patty be placed "forthwith" in an appropriate residential facility pursuant to her IEP. CPS was ordered to pay the costs of the placement that were not the legal responsibility of other agencies, such as the state department of education, state department of social services, the county education agency, and DMH. Furthermore, CPS was to apply, if necessary, to the county board of supervisors to approve or pay for this placement from the general county funds.

After this court order was issued, the director of CPS made a request to the county board of supervisors to fund or approve funds for

Patty's placement at Rehab Residential Center. However, the request never came before the board of supervisors. The chief administrative officer for the county, who had the power to determine funding issues that came before the board, decided not to do anything with the request. Consequently, no action was taken on it.

The county education agency administrators also decided to take no action related to the juvenile court order, which specified that this agency constituted Patty's school district of residence and, therefore, should pay for the school-related costs of Rehab Residential Center.

What Had Gone Wrong?

The fact that the request for funding for Patty's placement never came before the board of supervisors and that the county education agency ignored the juvenile court order was an indication of the weakness of the juvenile court in the state. The juvenile court had no power to call the respective agencies into court or to impose any sanctions on them. This weakness was detrimental to the well being of foster youth, over whom the court had tremendous authority and responsibility.

A Special Education Hearing

We decided we needed to take some further action to try to move this stymied process forward. Nancy and I filed a request for a special education hearing with the state special education hearing office (SEHO). Until now, we had been working with local county agencies. We now were bringing in the authority of SEHO, a state-contract agency whose decisions had clear authority over the local education agency.

Our purpose in doing this was to determine which educational agency was responsible for paying for the educational portion of Patty's residential program. We named all of the agencies we had been dealing with as parties to this hearing, including one new agency. We named the largest school district in the county as a party since there were some behind-the-scenes discussions with the attorney from the state department of education who argued that since the juvenile court was situated within the boundaries of this school district, and since the juvenile court had legal custody of Patty, that perhaps, this school district should be considered Patty's school district of residence. The fact that this school district was the largest in the county and had the "deepest pockets" was also mentioned in these discussions.

The Mediation

When a special education hearing is requested in the state where Patty lived, mediation is scheduled prior to the hearing in order to try to reach agreement on the issues. This is what had also occurred in Sharon's case.

The mediation for Patty was held in a conference room in the main headquarters of the largest school district in the county. The day we met for the mediation, the weather was sweltering and there was no air conditioning in the conference room. There were thirteen of us around the conference table, including the mediator from SEHO. The mediator on this case was one of the most skilled in the state. However, the mediators do not come to the mediations with awareness of the facts in the case. The purpose of the mediation is to try to set out the facts, the relevant law, and, hopefully, come to some agreement on the disputed issues. It was my job to review, for this group, the facts in Patty's case that brought us to the mediation. Shortly after my presentation, the mediator started meeting with each party separately to try to hammer out an agreement as to which educational agency would take responsibility for Patty. Even though we spent most of the day at this mediation trying to come to some agreement, it was to no avail. At the end of the day, we were no further advanced than when we had started. Consequently, we then specified in writing the issues for the administrative hearing, a procedure that follows mediation if agreement is not reached. The major issue was which educational agency is fiscally responsible for the provision of special education and related services for Patty?

A Political Solution

Before we had a chance to present our case to an administrative hearing officer from SEHO, however, Nancy's co-counsel, Rachael Woodman, decided to contact the state senator from the district in which her home was located to see if there was a political solution to funding Patty's placement in Rehab Residential Center. The timing was fortuitous. This state senator immediately contacted the state superintendent of education, one day before the state education budget was to be voted on in the state senate. The superintendent agreed to reimburse the largest school district in the county with state funds for the educational portion of Patty's stay at Rehab Residential Center. These funds for Patty then were specified in the state education budget. And this was how this school district came to be Patty's school district of residence.

Advocacy Considerations

Rachael Woodman was well acquainted with and had supported her state senator's election. This made it possible for her to ask for his help in working out funding arrangements for the residential program for Patty (see Exhibit 9.9).

A Placement IEP Meeting

Intervention

Once the school hurdle was overcome, things then fell into place fairly easily. Rehab Residential Center officially accepted Patty. Nancy attended an IEP meeting at the residential facility along with a representative from Patty's "new" school district of residence and the program head from DMH. All financial arrangements were specified on Patty's very comprehensive IEP.

The school district, where Rehab Residential Center was located, agreed to send a special education teacher to work on Patty's academic skills onsite at the head trauma facility. This teacher was to help her read a high interest/low vocabulary book at the third grade level and to read and follow simple directions. The teacher would also work

---

EXHIBIT 9.9.
Legislative Solutions

When other advocacy strategies fail to bring about important results for children, call upon your local and state legislators to help fashion solutions.

with her on telling time on an analog clock to the half hour and quarter hour and help her identify and state the value of common coins. Another mathematics objective was for Patty to do addition and subtraction using a calculator. For written language, the goal for Patty was to be able to compose and write a simple three-sentence paragraph with correct spelling and punctuation.

However, most of Patty's day would be taken up with services provided by head trauma specialists. A speech and language specialist would work with Patty on using a memory book so she would be able to follow a daily schedule and arrive on time at her many scheduled group activities throughout the day. The speech and language specialist also would work with Patty on maintaining the topic of conversation when talking with another person and also initiating conversation with staff, which was to include stating the staff person's name and the topic of conversation. In addition, this specialist would also help Patty learn to come up with alternative solutions to common problems.

An occupational therapist would spend time with Patty helping her initiate, follow through, and complete projects before beginning others. The occupational therapist also was to help her learn to ask for assistance when she did not understand a task.

The behavior therapist would help her respond appropriately without cursing, verbally abusing, or antagonizing others. A psychologist would work with her on monitoring and controlling her anxiety levels. This therapist would help Patty learn to ask for help when it was appropriate, set boundaries for herself and hold to them, and be assertive with others, which included telling them her needs.

A physical therapist would help Patty strengthen and increase the range of motion in her right leg. Her problems with her right leg were attributed to injuries related to her car accident. A nurse was to work with her on improving her level of independence in health-related areas, such as learning to identify her own medication and being able to take the appropriate medication under supervision. She also would learn to monitor and identify her need for health care and first aid.

A Six-Month IEP Review

As required by state law for students placed in residential facilities by DMH, an IEP meeting was held for Patty six months after her placement at Rehab Residential Center (Interagency Responsibilities for Related Services, 2004). All of the participants who attended her previous IEP meeting were again in attendance. At this meeting, plans were being made for Patty's transition to a less restrictive group home setting for head-injured adults that the Regional Center would be responsible for funding. Negotiations between DMH, the school district, and the Regional Center resulted in the Regional Center's acceptance of funding a group home placement for Patty upon her discharge from Rehab Residential Center. Since she was eighteen now, CPS was planning to terminate its jurisdiction of her.

Her IEP, at this time, described a young woman who had made progress at Rehab Residential Center. DMH noted significant progress in problem areas previously identified. She had not attempted to run away from the facility or engage in inappropriate sexual behavior. Her cognitive skills were reported to have improved to the eleven- to thirteen-year-old range. The biggest increase was seen in her judgment and her ability to deal with abstractions. Although, she still had moderate difficulty shifting from one cognitive task to another. She was described as moderately vulnerable to overstimulation and her social-emotional functioning was still below age level. However, she was less inclined to form superficial relationships and her ability to set limits was considered to be relatively good compared with same age peers without disabilities.

There had been no recent physical or verbal aggression in the residential setting, although, there was minimal verbal aggression in the school setting. However, she was described as being able to control her rude or antagonistic behavior 95 percent of the time at school and she was considered much improved at expressing anger appropriately. Patty was described as having normal competence relative to same-age peers in expressing emotions and describing her internal states. It was now felt she was able to understand the concept of resolving trauma rather than reenacting it. And she was said to be very good at forming a therapeutic alliance. Consequently, it was felt that she would continue to benefit from psychotherapy. Her coping strategies were considered to be age-appropriate. In addition, there was considerable improvement in her impulse control, which was now assessed at a thirteen- to fourteen-year-old level.

Advocacy Considerations

Plans were being made to transition Patty from the Rehab Residential Center to the group home that had been identified as appropriate for her. Nancy's role as Patty's attorney was to help her exit the foster care system in a way that would ensure she had a good, stable place to live and money to support her. The Regional Center was in place to fund Patty's group home and she also was set to receive Supplemental Security Insurance (SSI) from the Social Security Administration because of her disability.

CONCLUSION

When we saw how much progress Patty had made in six months at Rehab Residential Center, we felt vindicated in our struggle to have her placed there. However, one of the lessons we learned from the process was that the juvenile court was powerless to force the various agencies that had some responsibility for Patty to comply with the court order to fund her placement. Because of Patty's case, Advocacy Services embarked upon an effort through legislation to strengthen the power of the juvenile court in the state where Patty lived. This effort was ultimately successful, thus giving the juvenile court the authority to "join in the juvenile court proceedings any agency that the court determines has failed to meet a legal obligation to provide services to the minor" (*Juvenile Court Proceedings,* 2006) Prior to the passage of the legislation, one legislative committee noted: "the amendment addresses the needs of the most difficult-to-serve population of dependent children and wards of the court—children with multiple service needs [who are] legally entitled to services from several public agencies. The fact that multiple agencies are involved often results in a failure to provide legally mandated services: the buck gets passed from agency to agency without the child getting any services" (Senate Committee Report, 1992).

Why were we finally able to obtain the right services for Patty when, for many years, a number of agencies had not been able to properly educate her, resolve her mental health issues, or care for her? One answer is that we tried to find services to meet Patty's actual needs, rather than simply fitting her into the typical service options. We also used the available laws and did so creatively to try to achieve our ends. Our general principle was to try all avenues available and to pursue them vigorously. When we were stymied in our efforts with one agency, we tried another. We contested denials of services through administrative hearings using federal and state special education laws and state laws for services for individuals with developmental disabilities. We engaged the juvenile court to try to resolve the issue of which agencies were responsible for funding Patty's placement. We were determined to obtain the services that Patty needed and put in tremendous time and effort on her behalf. In the final analysis, however, it took political pressure to reach our goal for Patty's treatment.

SUMMARY

The purpose of this chapter was to highlight how a variety of laws could be used in attempting to arrange a higher level of funding required for the only residential placement in the state deemed appropriate for a foster youth whose special needs had never been adequately addressed. The chapter shows how difficult obtaining funding from a local education agency can be when a child does not have a parent and the laws are not clear about what constitutes the child's school district of residence. In addition, the chapter makes clear the difficulty of patching together funding from multiple agencies when the juvenile court lacks adequate legal authority to enforce court orders. Finally, the chapter illuminates how a political solution was used to work out the funding arrangements when other avenues were stymied or not progressing quickly enough.

Chapter 10

Anthony:
Advocating for Foster Home Placement

INTRODUCTION

Anthony, an African-American boy, had a difficult start in life. His mother neglected him because of her mental illness. She failed to feed him properly and, as a very young child, he was diagnosed with malnutrition. Later, his father was found to lack the necessary skills to care for him and he was removed from his custody. Because Anthony was nonverbal at the age of four and a half, mistakenly, he was considered to have severe mental retardation. As a result, he was placed in a group home with children who were very low functioning cognitively and did not receive the kind of ongoing stimulation and enrichment that he needed.

This chapter describes the advocacy efforts by Anthony's legal representatives to remove him from the group home that was counterproductive to his well-being, to place him in the home of a loving foster family, and to support the foster home placement. This support required finding an appropriate special education classroom for Anthony so that his foster mother was not being called constantly to come pick him up from school due to his misbehavior. Requiring his foster mother to be on call to pick him up during the school day had the very real potential of jeopardizing his foster home placement. It is this kind of circumstance, if not addressed adequately, that can lead one agency's failures (i.e., the school district) to destabilize the efforts of another agency (i.e., CPS) leaving an interagency crack through which foster children can, and often do, fall.

The Systematic Mistreatment of Children in the Foster Care System
© 2007 by The Haworth Press, Taylor & Francis Group. All rights reserved.
doi:10.1300/5136_10

What Anthony needed educationally was a special education classroom with a teacher who was skilled not only in developing his communication skills, but also was adept at setting up and carrying out a positive behavior management program for him. This combination was not easy to find. Anthony's case starkly reminds us that being an integral member of a nurturing family unit and having an appropriate school program can make the difference between failure and success for many children in the foster care system.

CASE STUDY OF ANTHONY

CPS Files a Petition

Child protective services (CPS) filed a petition with the juvenile court when Anthony was six months old alleging that his mother had limited ability to care for him because of her chronic and severe mental illness. Records noted that Anthony had prenatal exposure to marijuana and alcohol, although there was no indication that he experienced withdrawal symptoms at birth.

Prevention

Anthony was allowed to remain in his parents' home at that time with monitoring by a CPS social worker (see Exhibit 10.1).

Detention and Disposition

Six months later, when Anthony was one year old, CPS officially detained him, moving him to the emergency shelter. From there, he was hospitalized since there was serious concern about his health. He remained hospitalized for a month due to malnutrition and chronic *otitis media* (i.e., middle ear infection). Anthony remained out of his parents' home for six months.

CPS then decided to place Anthony back with his father, who now was living with his own mother, in the hope that the two of them could provide the support that Anthony needed. Anthony's mother was given only monitored visits with her son having been found unable to care for Anthony. She had been diagnosed with paranoid schizophrenia, with acute exacerbation.

EXHIBIT 10.1.
Placement History

Time Period	Placement	Maltreatment	School
6 mos.	Home of parents	Neglect	Not in school
1 yr.	Emergency Shelter		Not in school
1 yr. 6 mos.	Home of father	Neglect	Not in school
4 yrs.	Kramer group home		Nightingale Elem.
7 yrs. 6 mos.	Foster home		Not in school
7 yrs. 9 mos.	Foster home		Kennedy Elem.
8 yrs. 8 mos.	Foster home		98th St. Elem.
9 yrs. 8 mos.	Foster home		Evergreen Elem.

Elem. = Elementary School.

Anthony's father had his own problems. He had a bullet lodged in his leg and, as a result, was frequently in pain. However, because Anthony's father was living with his own mother, CPS felt, and the court agreed, that for the time being, there was enough watchful support in the home for Anthony to be placed there. Also living in the home was the father's brother who was thought to have autism. Anthony's CPS social worker, during her monitoring visits, found Anthony to be doing well in his father's care and described him as a happy, outgoing, and playful little boy.

Intervention

When Anthony was almost two and a half, the court ordered an evaluation of his mother's psychiatric condition. The psychiatrist who evaluated her determined that she required a consistent, long-term treatment program. As a result of this evaluation, Anthony's mother enrolled in counseling at a mental health clinic. However, six months later, when the social worker checked on how the counseling was going, she discovered that Anthony's mother had never attended any of the counseling sessions.

Prevention

At the six-month judicial review court hearing, the social worker reported that Anthony's mother had not been successful with her monitored visits with Anthony. When she visited Anthony at his grandmother's home, she would become disruptive and physically aggressive with the adults who lived there. Nevertheless, the judge issued an order maintaining the monitored visits but continued to restrict her from living with Anthony. At the time the court hearing took place, however, the court orders had little effect since the mother's whereabouts were unknown.

What Had Gone Wrong?

Why did the CPS social worker fail to check on whether Anthony's mother was attending her counseling sessions until right before the six-month review court hearing? Unfortunately, this too often is a common practice because of the extremely large caseloads of CPS social workers. Whether regular checking on his mother's attendance at her counseling sessions would have made a difference in her compliance is unclear. However, what was clear was that for Anthony's mother's psychiatric condition to be stabilized, it required compliance with her medication and regular psychiatric monitoring, which was not happening.

Concern about Anthony's Development

When Anthony was almost three, his social worker became concerned since she had never heard him speak actual words or sentences and, furthermore, he was not yet toilet trained. She had only heard Anthony make sounds that she described as gibberish.

Intervention

In looking back at a medical report when Anthony was six months, and at the emergency shelter, his social worker realized that the doctor, at that time, thought Anthony was developmentally delayed. Based on her current concerns about Anthony's development and the early medical report of his delay, the social worker decided to refer Anthony to the Regional Center for a determination of whether he currently had a developmental disability that would make him eligible for Regional Center services. The social worker also referred the father to a parenting class to improve his parenting skills and to a respite program for Anthony—a program that would provide childcare for Anthony and give his family some time away from him. Unfortunately, the respite program would not take Anthony because he was not toilet-trained and the father started, but never completed, the parenting class.

At age four and a half, a year and a half after the social worker's referral, Anthony's Regional Center evaluation described him as having a history, behavior, and cognitive skills consistent with autism. The evaluator, however, made clear that the results should be viewed with caution because of Anthony's history of deprivation and that he should be reevaluated when he was in a stable environment and after having attended school.

The evaluator based his conclusion about Anthony having autism on many factors—at four and a half he still was nonverbal, had low scores on tests of cognitive ability (between sixteen and twenty-nine months and he was sixty-six months at the time), and was not able to interact with other children or play with toys appropriately. In addition, he had poor concentration and attention; was overly active; physically aggressive; stubborn; destroyed property; engaged in excessive or peculiar preoccupations; and displayed unusual mannerisms, such as rocking back and forth. The recommendations were for Anthony to be placed in a highly structured school setting that stressed attention to tasks and language development and in a group home specializing in the care of children with developmental disabilities.

What Had Gone Wrong?

It took over a year for the Regional Center to diagnose Anthony's disabilities and make him eligible for Regional Center Services. State law requires that evaluations be completed within sixty to 120 days. The sixty-day timeline is required if a delay would "harm the mental or physical development of the person or cause imminent risk of placement in a more restrictive setting" (Lanterman Development Disabilities Services Act, 1969).

Advocacy Considerations

The CPS social worker could have filed a complaint with the state department of developmental services when she realized that Anthony's evaluation was not being completed within legal timelines.

Removal from His Father's Home

Prevention

One month after Anthony's Regional Center diagnosis, when he was four years and seven months, based on the CPS social worker's recommendation, the court ordered that Anthony be removed from his father's home; although, it took an additional two months before Anthony actually was removed. The social worker indicated in her detention report that Anthony's father had tried to care for his son, but he was limited in his ability and lacked necessary skills. She wrote that he needed counseling to help him understand Anthony's problems, including how to care for and discipline his son. The report also stated that Anthony's mother had chronic paranoid schizophrenia and, at that time, was incarcerated for burglary.

Intervention

Almost two months later, Anthony was placed in the Kramer Group Home for children with developmental disabilities and enrolled in a preschool program at a special education school, called Nightingale, in the local school district. Anthony's father was ordered by the court to visit his son frequently, to attend counseling, and to participate in a Regional Center program to learn how to cope with his son's behavior and to discipline him appropriately. As it turned out, his father did not follow through on these orders.

Inconsistent Evaluation Reports

When Anthony was five years and one month, which was three months after placement at the Kramer Group Home, a psychologist diagnosed him as having severe mental retardation after having tested his cognitive, academic, self-help, and perceptual-motor skills. The psychologist noted that Anthony was only able to say isolated words, such as "yes," "no," and "water." He also reported that the caregiver at the group home told him that Anthony did not have any behavior problems, but that he seemed quiet and almost fearful.

Six months later, the school district psychologist, having completed an extensive evaluation of Anthony, criticized previous evaluations of his cognitive ability for not using a language-free assessment given his extreme delay in expressive language. Rather than finding severe mental retardation, this psychologist found Anthony's cognitive abilities (excluding expressive language) to only be slightly delayed, at the low normal level of functioning. Anthony was five years and seven months and his cognitive performance was assessed at the four and a half to five-year-old level.

The school psychologist assessed Anthony on the Childhood Autism Rating Scale and found that he displayed some characteristics consistent with autism, but did not exhibit the array of required characteristics to a definitive degree. He described Anthony as having high energy levels interspersed with periods of lethargy and staring into space. He exhibited inappropriate emotional responses, abnormal expressive language including making peculiar noises, and echolalia (compulsive repetition of the words spoken by another). In addition, the psychologist indicated that Anthony engaged in significant acting out, attention-seeking behaviors, which often required one-to-one intervention. He also described him as having very limited ability in general to remain task-oriented. The recommendations by this psychologist were for an in-depth observation and assessment of Anthony's language functioning and consideration for placement in a language-intensive school program.

A month later, when Anthony was five years and eight months, the school district's speech and language specialist evaluated Anthony and found his comprehension to be delayed by at least two years. At the time, he was able to follow a one-step direction. His expressive language was severely delayed in all areas—morphology, syntax, semantics, and pragmatics.

What Had Gone Wrong?

Anthony, along with all the other children whose stories are described in this book, had numerous psychological assessments requested usually by their social workers or by their foster or group home caretakers. Some of these assessments were done extremely well by highly skilled assessors; however, too many, unfortunately, were cursory assessments using tests that were inappropriate for the child but, nevertheless, led to a diagnosis with placement ramifications. Anthony was a prime example of the costs to a child of inappropriate assessment. He had been placed in a group home with children with severe cognitive delays and ended up imitating the behavior of the other children, making it appear that he was significantly more delayed than he really was (see Exhibit 10.2).

Permanency Planning Hearing

At the next court hearing, the decision was to continue Anthony in foster care, thus making long-term foster care as Anthony's permanent placement plan. He also was to remain in the Kramer group home with other children with severe developmental delays. The social worker's report for the court hearing indicated that Anthony was now talking more without simply echoing what others were saying. He could say, "Want to go to bathroom," "want to eat," and "waiting for bus." The social worker noted that Anthony had been unable to say any of these phrases the previous year. He also was toilet-trained now.

School Placement

An IEP meeting, held for Anthony when he was almost six, identified him as eligible for special education services on the basis of a specific learning disability. The decision of the team was for him to be placed in a full-day special education class in the same special

---

EXHIBIT 10.2.
Assessment

Ensure that assessment instruments used are appropriate, assessors are qualified, and that the assessments are sufficiently comprehensive to accurately describe the child. Seek additional assessments if a diagnosis seems suspect.

education school where he had been attending preschool. The reason for this segregated placement, solely with children with disabilities, was that, according to his IEP, a "regular education campus cannot provide for . . . [his] need for close adult supervision and specialized services." His IEP identified the following required services: language and speech services, once a week for thirty minutes, and adapted physical education, twice a week for a total of sixty minutes.

A little over a year later at another IEP meeting, when Anthony had just turned seven, the IEP team, in addition to identifying him as having a specific learning disability, added a language and speech disability to his IEP. His school placement, however, remained the same along with his language and speech and adapted physical education services. This IEP noted, however, that Anthony's language skills had improved and that he was no longer throwing tantrums at the group home.

What Had Gone Wrong?

Why was Anthony placed on a segregated special education school site when the IDEA (2004) specifically requires children with disabilities to be placed in the least restrictive school environment? The specialized services that Anthony required—language and speech services for thirty minutes per week and adapted physical education for sixty minutes per week—were available on most general education campuses in the school district. The school district, unfortunately, had a practice of placing many students with disabilities on segregated school campuses even though many of them would have been able to function just fine in a special education class on a general education campus (see Exhibit 10.3).

EXHIBIT 10.3.
Least Restrictive Environment

Least restrictive environment refers to the requirement that students with disabilities must participate and be educated with students without disabilities to the maximum extent appropriate. (IDEA, 2004)

Resistance to Change of Home Placement

It had become clear that Anthony was much higher functioning than were the other children in the group home. The problem for Anthony of remaining in this home was that he was not getting the intellectual and language stimulation he needed and was imitating the behavior of the other children. Consequently, his social worker wanted to move him into a foster home with higher functioning children. However, the social worker faced resistance to the move by the owner of the group home.

Nancy, at Advocacy Services, having recently been appointed by the juvenile court to represent Anthony, went to visit him at his group home and agreed with the social worker that this setting was not in his best interests. She decided to talk with the supervising social worker on Anthony's case to see if she could help bring about a change of placement for him. What Nancy learned from this supervisor was that the owner of the group home had complained to higher-level administrators within CPS about Anthony's potential change of placement. And because of these complaints, the administrators were requiring that a strong case be made by his social worker before a change of placement could occur. Nancy then talked with the administrators at CPS about the case and the serious problems with this group home for Anthony. The administrators finally agreed with the need for the change of placement and the group home owner was made to understand why Anthony's placement should be changed, and it was then he was moved to a foster home.

Advocacy Considerations

When Nancy was appointed to represent Anthony, she established a positive relationship with his CPS social worker and, consequently, learned that the social worker had serious reservations about the group home where Anthony was residing. Nancy then visited Anthony in the group home to evaluate the placement for herself. When she was convinced that this group home placement was not in Anthony's best interest, she tried to bring about a change of placement by convincing high-level administrators within CPS that Anthony's current placement was not appropriate. Nancy, as Anthony's court-appointed attorney and also being well thought of within the child welfare community, was able to convince CPS administrators that Anthony did indeed need to be placed in a foster home. The fact that an opening was available with a skilled and nurturing foster mother also made Nancy's advocacy easier.

Foster Home Placement

Intervention

CPS removed Anthony from the group home and placed him in a home with foster parents. He was moved into his new foster home at the end of June. The foster parents, Angela and George, had two children of their own and four foster children for whom they cared. A summer law student, Kathy, working with Nancy at Advocacy Services, visited Anthony in his foster home. She reported that Anthony said he was happy in his new home. Kathy's observation was that the house was clean and the children seemed well cared for. Angela was out at the time Kathy visited and had left five of the children with a hired staff person, whom the law student found to be friendly and engaging. George was at work at his job at the fire department.

Later that day, Kathy talked with Angela who said that Anthony was not yet in school because his social worker had misplaced the papers needed to enroll him. After contacting the social worker and others at CPS, Kathy realized that they did not have Anthony's current IEP, which the new school was requiring before enrolling Anthony. Consequently, Kathy got in touch with the school that Anthony last had attended and requested that the records be forwarded to his new school immediately. Anthony's school records, including his IEP, promptly arrived and his foster mother then was able to enroll him in school.

What Had Gone Wrong?

The problem of foster youths being out of school for long periods of time when they change home placements occurs all too frequently. What happens is that the new home is not within the boundaries of the school or school district the student has been attending, thus requiring a change of school placement. Concern about this issue has led to state legislation (AB 490, 2003) that requires school districts to allow children in the foster care system to remain in the same school, even when their home placement changes. If, however, it is in the child's best interest to change schools, the child is to be enrolled immediately, even if he or she does not have all pertinent school and health records at the time of enrollment. This legislation is described more fully in the last chapter of this book.

School Placement Change

Intervention

In the fall, three months before Anthony's eighth birthday, his school placement was changed. He was moved to a full-day special education class for students with learning disabilities located on a regular education elementary school campus.

I became involved in Anthony's case several months later when his foster mother had become increasingly concerned that his classroom placement was not at all meeting his needs. Angela called Nancy to share her concerns about Anthony's school placement. She told her that she had talked with the school psychologist, hoping to convince her that Anthony was not appropriately placed in his current classroom and that he needed to be moved to a different type of classroom placement. But Angela said she had not made any progress in bringing about a change of classroom placement for Anthony.

Nancy had told Angela that I would contact her and make arrangements to observe Anthony at school. When I called her, she told me that Anthony's teacher called her several times a week and, sometimes, even daily insisting that she pick Anthony up from school because he was misbehaving. She then would have to stop whatever she was doing and drive to the school to get Anthony and take him home. At other times, she said, the teacher called her during the school day so she could talk with Anthony on the telephone to tell him to stop doing whatever misbehavior the teacher reported he was engaged in.

Angela was convinced that Anthony was not in the proper school placement if he was being sent home as frequently as he was and if she always had to be on call to attend to his misconduct. I too was concerned with the facts Angela was reporting, since Anthony's classroom placement should have included enough structure and support so that his behavioral problems would be addressed as part of his individualized special education program. I further was concerned that there never was any paperwork (such as suspension notices) that accompanied Anthony being sent home from school and, consequently, there was no written record of the problems. I told Angela that I would take a look at Anthony's classroom, talk to the teacher, and see how Anthony was functioning in that setting. Then we could decide on how to proceed.

I called the teacher, John Anderson, and set up a time to come and observe the classroom. On the morning we had arranged, I arrived at the school at twenty minutes after nine and, after checking in at the main office, made my way up to Anthony's classroom on the second floor. Upon entering the classroom, Mr. Anderson acknowledged my presence with a nod and motioned for me to take a seat near his desk, which put me close enough to what was happening in the classroom, but not so close that my presence would interfere with the teaching or learning activities.

The classroom was set up with tables and chairs in two different corners of the room so the teacher and his classroom aide could each work independently with a small group of students. The central area in the classroom was carpeted and empty of any tables or chairs; students could sit in a circle there on the floor. There were low bookshelves along two sides of the carpeted space that held games, books, and other materials for the students to use.

I counted twelve students in the classroom along with the teacher and his aide. Four students were working with Mr. Anderson, four other students were working with the aide, and the remaining four students were doing independent activities such as puzzles and coloring. Anthony was by himself on the floor diligently arranging and re-arranging Popsicle sticks into block-shaped numbers. He looked small and thin compared to the other students. After awhile, Anthony left the classroom without asking permission (presumably to use the bathroom) and returned a short time later.

Mr. Anderson then called Anthony over to join five other students sitting around a table. After reviewing facts about Frederick Douglas' life while showing the students pictures of Douglas in a book, Mr. Anderson asked the students to draw their own pictures about

Frederick Douglas' life and tell him three sentences about their pictures. As the students described their pictures, Mr. Anderson wrote down what they said. The students then were to copy the sentences on their papers on the lines under their pictures.

All the students except Anthony were able to do the assignment. While Mr. Anderson was reviewing facts about Douglas' life and showing pictures of him, Anthony did not seem to be paying attention. When asked, Anthony was unable to tell Mr. Anderson anything about Frederick Douglas' life.

After the Frederick Douglas activity, the aide took the students out on the yard for recess and I had an opportunity to talk with Mr. Anderson. He told me that Anthony's learning problems and behaviors were significantly different from those of the other students in the class. While he described Anthony's strengths as reading (primer level) and math (first-grade level), he said that Anthony's particular needs made it difficult for him to function well in this classroom. He described Anthony as not appearing to understand most oral language. Consequently, he could not follow through consistently when given a one-step direction verbally. He said Anthony primarily used one-word sentences, although Mr. Anderson felt he was capable of putting together longer sentences. Given Anthony's poor language ability, it was not surprising that, Mr. Anderson reported, he did not have any friends in the class and could not interact appropriately with his peers. Mr. Anderson said Anthony frequently touched other students, even though he was told he was to keep his hands to himself. While Mr. Anderson felt Anthony could in fact learn the routines in games, nevertheless, he was unable to engage in appropriate turn taking without teacher assistance and he could not teach the rules of a game to another child.

Mr. Anderson went on to describe what he called Anthony's particularly unusual behaviors. He said that about every couple of weeks Anthony would make animal noises and crawl around on the floor. He also described him as very single-minded, doing the same activity over and over, and it was difficult for him to move from an activity in which he was engaged to a different activity. According to Mr. Anderson, Anthony was extremely uncooperative when there was a substitute teacher. He relayed that Anthony said the daily Pledge of Allegiance in a loud monotone voice, generally had a flat affect, and did not seem to laugh spontaneously. He also described Anthony as always drawing the same thing—a sun and rain—in the pictures the teacher had the students draw after reading them a new story, no matter what the content of the story was. Mr. Anderson felt that Anthony needed a classroom with fewer students in order to learn how to interact appropriately with others and to improve his overall behavior.

After my visitation in Anthony's classroom, I called the school psychologist to discuss my observations with her. I told her how often Anthony was being sent home from school, reminded her that these were inappropriate suspensions from school, let her know the concerns that Mr. Anderson had about that classroom placement for Anthony, and said that his foster mother wanted an IEP meeting to discuss appropriate classroom placement for Anthony. I also discussed with the school psychologist Anthony's need for a classroom placement where language development was a strong focus of the classroom and the teacher had appropriate training in this area. The school psychologist said there had to be a reassessment of Anthony in order to make the kind of placement change I was recommending.

School District Assessment and IEP Meeting

The school district reevaluated Anthony, who was now in the second grade. The school psychologist found Anthony to be functioning in the range of low average to average in his cognitive ability, but also cautioned that his true cognitive ability could not yet be determined due to multiple factors (i.e., language delay, distractibility). She found, however, that he grasped new concepts quickly.

Anthony's academic achievement also was tested. He was found to be at the prefirst-grade level in both reading and spelling, but at the end of the first grade level in arithmetic. He required adult direction to complete most academic tasks and was easily distracted, even in a one-to-one setting. He needed reminders to continue to focus on the task at hand. The psychologist found Anthony to be a likeable, friendly child who was eager to please and sensitive to the needs of others.

The speech and language specialist evaluated Anthony's skills and found he had a significant language delay/disorder in all language areas. His comprehension difficulties significantly interfered with his ability to converse and respond to tasks appropriately. The speech and language specialist recommended that Anthony be placed in a full-day special education class for students with aphasia (i.e., a language disorder).

Once the assessments of Anthony were completed, the IEP meeting should have been held soon after. However, this did not happen. So I called the school psychologist to find out why the IEP meeting had not been scheduled. While I never learned specifically what had caused the delay, soon after my call, the IEP meeting was scheduled.

At the IEP meeting, the psychologist and speech and language specialist reported on their assessment findings. Based on the assessment by the speech and language specialist, there was agreement that Anthony required a change of placement to a class for students with aphasia. In addition, counseling, once a week for a thirty-minute session, was added to his IEP in order to help him identify his feelings of anger and frustration and use more appropriate ways of expressing those feelings. Anthony also was to receive adapted physical education twice a week for a total of sixty minutes.

What Had Gone Wrong?

Although we did not find out specifically why an IEP meeting for Anthony had not been scheduled within legal timelines, it was general knowledge that many district psychologists were overwhelmed with the numbers of children for whom assessments and IEP meetings were required. Consequently, many cases, including Anthony's, were out of compliance with special education legal timelines.

Advocacy Considerations

I called the school psychologist when I realized Anthony's IEP meeting had not been scheduled and the timelines had been exceeded. My phone call was successful and the IEP meeting was scheduled immediately. Had that not occurred, there were legal options I would have taken, such as filing a noncompliance complaint or for a special education due process hearing to force the district to schedule the IEP meeting (see Exhibit 10.4).

EXHIBIT 10.4.
Special Education Time Lines

When it appears that special education time lines will be exceeded, contact the special education administrator and indicate your concern about the time line violation. If this strategy does not obtain the desired results, you might choose to file a noncompliance complaint with the appropriate state or federal agency.

Change of School Placement

Intervention

Anthony's placement at Evergreen Elementary School in Ms. De Champ's class for children with language disorders occurred at the end of the summer prior to his third grade school year. It was four months before Anthony's ninth birthday. Ms. De Champ initially had concerns about Anthony's hyperactivity. Once he started receiving medication during the school day to control his hyperactivity, Ms. De Camp found him easier to handle, although his attention span still was extremely short and his academic skills were below those of the other students in the class.

In October, about two months after he was placed in Ms. De Champ's class, I contacted her to set up an observation. During our phone conversation, she told me that Anthony was progressing well and, at that time, fitting in beautifully in her class. He, however, still needed considerable one-to-one attention to understand assignments and to remain focused on an assigned task. To help with this problem, the school intended to find an older student to serve as a peer tutor for Anthony for two hours each day. We agreed on a day and time for me to observe Anthony in class.

I arrived at the school at 10:45 a.m. on the designated day of my observation. Including Anthony, there were eight boys in the class with Ms. De Champ and a full-time classroom aide. Several of the boys seemed to have not only language problems, but also were quite active and seemed to have problems keeping their hands to themselves, listening when others were speaking, and generally following directions. When I arrived, the class was involved in a language lesson. There were ten words written on the chalkboard (e.g., game, garden, book, boy, dog). Ms. De Champ selected one of the words and asked a child to make a sentence with the word without using the word "I." When it was Anthony's turn, Ms. De Champ asked him to make a sentence using the word "dog." Anthony said, "We have a dog." Ms. De Champ then asked Anthony if he really had a dog at home. When he said "yes," she asked him what color the dog was. Anthony promptly said "yellow" and Ms. De Champ told him to say, "We have a yellow dog," which Anthony did. Ms. De Champ continued to ask Anthony questions about the dog, such as, its name and size, and then had Anthony include the dog's name and its size in his sentence. I was quite pleased thinking that Anthony may have found an appropriate placement. He appeared significantly more aware of what was going on in the classroom than when I had observed him in his previous school. It was, however, still clear that he required one-to-one attention to understand what the teacher was asking him to do. He was able to stay seated at his desk, but he appeared quite fidgety, swinging his feet back and forth under it and constantly touching and moving things on the top of his desk.

When the students went out to recess with the aide, I had an opportunity to talk briefly with Ms. De Champ. She relayed that the school had found a peer tutor for Anthony who worked with him for forty-five minutes daily during reading. She felt the one-to-one attention worked extremely well for him and that Anthony would benefit significantly from a full-time one-to-one aide on a daily basis. Ms. De Champ was convinced that Anthony had the ability to function well in her largely academic class. However, he needed significant help not only to stay focused on his class assignments but also to understand what was being asked of him and what was going on in class.

Overall, I thought this class, with its strong focus on language development, was quite appropriate and that Anthony would benefit from being in it. However, I did have some concerns about the teacher. While she seemed to have good rapport with Anthony and genuinely appeared to care about him, she had a somewhat negative and punitive manner in disciplining and setting limits for the students.

Meeting with the School Psychologist

After my classroom observation, I went to meet with the school psychologist with whom I had earlier set up a meeting. Anthony's IEP counseling goals were for him to develop friends and communicate concerns, thoughts, and feelings appropriately to peers. The school psychologist told me that she met with Anthony weekly for thirty to forty-five minute sessions. In the initial sessions, she said Anthony had trouble following directions and was unable to participate in a conversation due to what she thought to be his severe deficits in listening and comprehending. Overall, however, she felt that Anthony was making continuous progress. Since she first started counseling him, his on-task behavior had increased from two to three minutes to sometimes as long as twenty minutes, depending on the activity. Initially, Anthony had difficulty sharing materials with a classmate, grabbing and hording them instead. He now was better able to share, was doing better at "turn-taking," and was beginning to use words to let a classmate know what he wanted. He was able to make and maintain eye contact with the school psychologist and was learning how to do that with peers as well.

Request for a One-to-One Aide

An IEP meeting was scheduled about a month after I had observed Anthony in class. I arrived at the meeting to discover that Ms. De Champ was the only other person in attendance. Ms. De Champ explained that the school psychologist, who was to be the administrator designee at the meeting, had written her a note saying that she had to test a student and therefore could not attend. Anthony's foster mother had called at the last minute to say she could not attend but that the meeting could proceed without her. I faced a dilemma at that moment. I was aware we did not have a legally constituted IEP meeting, but I decided to proceed with the meeting anyway.

Ms. De Champ discussed with me and noted on the IEP that Anthony's behavior had improved considerably after he started receiving a dose of medication to curb his hyperactivity during the school day. She also indicated that he was not at all aggressive and was respectful of adults. She described Anthony's academic functioning as being at a high kindergarten level, but that he had great difficulty comprehending what was said to him. This difficulty with comprehension particularly affected his ability to follow directions given for classroom assignments as well as to complete his schoolwork. He had to be told at least twice and sometimes four times how to complete each section on a given assignment. After discussions with Ms. De Champ about what she felt would aid Anthony's functioning in class and from my own observations, I requested a one-to-one aide for Anthony and asked Ms. De Champ to write my request on the IEP.

Advocacy Considerations

A legally constituted IEP meeting minimally requires that there be in attendance a school administrator, a special education teacher or service provider, a regular education teacher if the child is in or might be in regular education, and the child's parent. If assessment information is to be discussed, there must be a school district representative capable of interpreting it. Obviously, this meeting was far from the legal requirements. So why did I continue with it being aware that it was not legally constituted?

Since I was representing Anthony's foster mother and she had given approval to go ahead with the meeting in her absence, I felt it was in Anthony's best interest to continue with this meeting and try to obtain the services he needed in order to function well. I knew that if we postponed this meeting, it would take several weeks to set up another one. I also knew that his foster mother had to sign the IEP before it could be implemented, so she would have an opportunity to disagree with any part of it if she so chose. Finally, since it was not Anthony's fault that the school district had not sent an administrator to the meeting, I strongly felt that he should not be penalized by this violation of the law. I knew from my discussions with Ms. De Champ that the only way to get an aide specifically designated for Anthony was to request it on his IEP. Ms. De Champ had been trying to obtain additional help in the classroom for Anthony but, other than the minimal amount of time with a peer tutor, she had been unsuccessful. I felt this might move things along.

Further Advocacy Efforts to Obtain a One-to-One Aide

I talked with Angela Bolton, Anthony's foster mother, after the IEP meeting to let her know what had occurred. She still was very much in agreement that Anthony should receive a one-to-one aide in the classroom.

About a week later, however, Ms. De Champ informed me that she had just learned that all the aide positions in the district were "frozen" and no additional aides would be hired. After discussing the case with Nancy and Ms. Bolton, I decided to file for a due process hearing to try to obtain the aide we all felt Anthony needed if he were to make educational progress. I drafted a letter to the state special education hearing office (SEHO) requesting a mediation prior to the hearing to try to resolve the issue (see Exhibit 10.5).

Several days after filing for the hearing and mediation, I spoke with Ms. De Champ. She told me that the school district program specialist, who was over the special education classes in her region, told her to write up a more extensive justification for a one-to-one aide for Anthony than currently appeared in his IEP. Ms. De Champ said she planned to do that and would send me a copy, which she did within the next couple of days. Her memo stated:

1. Even with proper medication, Anthony cannot sit alone and start a task even after having been instructed on how to do it.
2. He is extremely low in the area of comprehension, needs multiple examples by someone sitting right next to him in order to comprehend, has difficulty in transferring verbal knowledge to a written task, and will say "I can't do it" when given a written assignment.
3. Most of the time, his medication deters any severe behavior problems in class; but, at times, he still is extremely hyperactive and someone must sit right next to him so that he can function.

EXHIBIT 10.5.
File for a Special Education Hearing

When it is clear that requested special education services are not forthcoming and you have exhausted routine avenues for attaining the services, file for a special education hearing. Use the mediation process prior to the hearing to attain the services and negotiate your differences with the school district.

After I received Ms. De Champ's memo, I contacted her to see whether it had any effect on securing an aide for Anthony. She told me that the coordinator of special education had met with her and communicated that district policy only allowed for assigning a one-to-one aide for a child when the child exhibits aggressive behavior. This information did not bode well for Anthony, even though such a policy (although unwritten) would appear to be a violation of the IDEA.

Advocacy Considerations

The IDEA (2004) requires that the educational program of a special education student be individually designed to meet the student's unique needs. Consequently, the school district must determine what the particular needs of a given child with a disability are rather than having a blanket policy denying specific services to students with specific disabilities or behavior characteristics.

Special Education Mediation

The mediation was held a couple weeks after my conversation with Ms. De Champ. A mediator from SEHO was assigned to help mediate the case. We met in one of the regional offices of the school district. Nancy and I attended along with Anthony's foster mother. On behalf of the school district, those in attendance were the coordinators of special education and psychological services and Ms. De Champ. I presented the issues in the case and the district administrators each read reports, one from the school psychologist at Anthony's school and the other from a behavior specialist who had observed Anthony in Ms. De Champ's class. I was not surprised that the school psychologist did not support a full-time one-to-one aide for Anthony. The behavior specialist made several recommendations, which included that Anthony receive ongoing teacher supervision throughout the day, but did not specifically recommend a one-to-one aide. I was surprised when Ms. De Champ forcefully made her case for Anthony's need for one-to-one assistance; since, in my experience, teachers often were intimidated in front of school district administrators. Ms. De Champ explained that neither she nor her classroom assistant could provide the one-to-one attention that Anthony required and still attend to the needs of the other children in the class. After Ms. De Champ's report, there was a discussion of how Anthony had fared with some peer tutors and the extent to which he was making progress toward his IEP goals.

The coordinator of special education readily agreed to provide one-to-one assistance for Anthony, but was adamant against hiring an aide to provide this service. His solution was that Anthony would be provided the one-to-one assistance by either a peer tutor or an adult volunteer. Ms. De Champ relayed that Anthony had done well with a student who had provided peer tutoring for a two-week period for forty-five minute sessions daily. However, the new peer tutor, who had worked with Anthony briefly, while having considerable patience, was not as quick in catching on to how to work best with him. I was skeptical of the peer tutor or adult volunteer solution believing that Anthony needed someone who was trained and who would be a consistent presence.

At that point, in the mediation, the mediator had us focus on the specific times in the school day when Ms. De Champ felt that Anthony absolutely needed one-to-one assistance. She narrowed the timeslots to 9:00 to 9:45 a.m., 10:10 to 10:45 a.m., and 1:15 to 2:00 p.m., those times in the school day requiring sustained attention to academic instruction and some independent academic work.

I raised the question that if we were to agree to a peer tutor or adult volunteer, how could we be sure that a tutor or volunteer would be available during the times Ms. De Champ specified that Anthony needed the one-to-one assistance the most. The coordinator of special education said that the school outreach coordinator would be assigned to recruit the tutor or volunteer aide and would work with Ms. De Champ in selecting someone.

The concern that I then raised was that the tutor or volunteer aide would likely not have experience in working with a student such as Anthony or in providing one-to-one assistance. I argued that in order for us to agree to this arrangement, there would have to be some training built in for the tutor or volunteer aide. I was gratified when the coordinator of special education offered to have both a district program specialist and a behavior specialist provide consultation to Ms. De Champ and the person or persons providing the assistance for Anthony. They would observe the classroom on a weekly basis, write reports of their observations, and provide training to those who were providing the one-to-one assistance. The coordinator of special education agreed to include a date in the mediation agreement when all of this would be in place. We also specified in the agreement that the mediation would again convene in three weeks either by phone or in person, depending on how the plan was progressing and its effectiveness.

I left the mediation with mixed feelings about whether our agreement would provide Anthony the support that he needed. I was glad that the program and behavior specialists would be observing the class and providing consultation to both Ms. De Champ and the person who would be assisting Anthony. I thought the specialists actually might help Ms. De Champ shore up her classroom management strategies. But I also worried that using a peer tutor or volunteer aide rather than a paid individual specifically hired to work with Anthony would not provide the consistency and experience that Anthony needed. Nevertheless, I figured it was worth a try and we always had the option of going to a hearing if the plan did not work out. By the time we signed an interim agreement, the only people left in the room were the mediator, the two school administrators, and I. Ms. De Champ had to go back to her classroom; Angela Bolton had to go care for her children; and Nancy had another meeting to attend.

Advocacy Considerations

Why did I agree to an interim mediation agreement about which I had reservations? First, it is important to understand that the agreement was an interim, and not a final, agreement. If the plan did not work out, I could recommend that Anthony's foster mother not sign a final agreement and then we could proceed to a hearing to try to obtain a full-time one-to-one aide for Anthony.

Second, Anthony had been successful with a peer tutor. I now had to see whether the district could find peer tutors or volunteer aides to cover the hours they were needed and whether with training, they could be effective with Anthony.

Third, I was aware of the concern, in the research literature, that indicated that some students became overly dependent on their one-to-one aides (Giangreco, Edelman, Luiselli, & MacFarland, 1997; Marks, Schrader, & Levine, 1999). Because of this, I thought there might be some worth in using several different people to assist Anthony if, in fact, they were adequately trained.

And finally, I thought if Ms. De Champ could improve her behavior management techniques, it was possible that Anthony would not need quite as much one-to-one assistance.

Second Mediation

Three weeks after our first mediation took place a second mediation was scheduled as a telephone conference. I learned during this phone conference that, as of the previous day, two student tutors and an adult volunteer were providing one-to-one assistance to Anthony during the specified times of the school day. In addition, the program specialist was observing the class twice a week and providing consultation and the behavior specialist was doing so once a week. The behavior specialist had determined that Anthony's instructional program should be divided into seven-minute blocks, since Anthony was not able to concentrate on academic tasks longer.

During the conference call, I raised the question of what would occur if one of the tutors or the adult volunteer were absent. The district agreed to have the school outreach coordinator make sure to replace the peer tutor or volunteer in case of their absence.

We ended the phone conference by scheduling an IEP meeting a month later with mediation to follow.

Classroom Observations

Prior to the IEP meeting, I scheduled two classroom observations to get a sense of how Anthony was faring in the classroom with the system of one-to-one assistance that we had put in place. I arrived at the classroom about 1:00 p.m. Ms. De Champ met with me briefly informing me that it had been helpful for Anthony having the peer tutors. However, she said that she had found it somewhat difficult because there had not been consistency with the tutors—there had been six already—and each time there was a change, she had to train the new person. I asked her how the changes were affecting Anthony and she indicated that it did not seem to matter to Anthony who the person was who was assisting him.

Ms. De Champ described the procedure that the behavior specialist recommended for Anthony's assistants to use with him. She called it "Praise, Prompt, and Leave." Ms. De Champ felt that the Praise, Prompt, and Leave approach (Jones, 2007) was helpful with Anthony, but it was difficult to implement consistently because of the change of tutors (see Exhibit 10.6).

One of Anthony's one-to-one peer tutors was assisting Anthony during my observation. This tutor seemed to be following the Prompt, Praise, and Leave strategy fairly successfully, although there were times when Anthony appeared to need additional instruction. He was able to remain on task only for short periods of time, but could be redirected back to the task by the tutor.

The second time I observed the classroom was in the morning and Anthony had a hard time attending to the class instruction. He seemed unable to concentrate or listen to the lesson that Ms. De Champ was presenting to the class. The student peer tutor was sitting right next to Anthony, but had little positive effect on his behavior. Ms. De Champ

---

EXHIBIT 10.6.
Praise, Prompt, and *Leave*

This strategy has three steps: *Praise* for work well done, *Prompt* on what to correct or do next and assurance that the instructor will be back soon to check further progress, and then *Leave* to give time to the student to make necessary corrections or to continue working. The total time for PPL is about 30 seconds to one minute per student. It is not intended to provide in-depth instruction, but rather a mid-course correction that includes reinforcement and guidance.

Praise—Approach the student with specific honest praise.
    Example: "The one's column is added correctly."
Prompt—Evaluate the problem and provide a guiding prompt.
    Example: "Double check the 10's column."
Leave—Assure the student that you will be back and move on to the next student.
    Example: "I will be back in a minute to see how you are doing."

Praise, Prompt, and *Leave* is a strategy from *Fred Jones Tools for Teaching.* Second Edition. (2007). Santa Cruz, CA. www.fredjones.com.

expressed concern to me about what to do with Anthony on the days he was extremely hyperactive and had difficulty maintaining focus and attention.

IEP Meeting and Third Mediation

About a month after our telephone conference, an individualized education program (IEP) meeting was held for Anthony with the mediator present. The program and behavior specialists reported on their observations of Anthony in the classroom and their consultation with Ms. De Champ and the classroom one-to-one assistants. Ms. De Champ described how Anthony was progressing and shared her concern about his hyperactivity and difficulty in paying attention on certain mornings. The behavior specialist agreed to work with Ms. De Champ on strategies to help Anthony when he was particularly hyperactive and distractible. Some new goals and objectives were added to Anthony's IEP as well as a delineation of the one-to-one assistance he was receiving.

After the IEP meeting, the coordinators of special education and psychological services arrived for the mediation. We drafted another interim mediation agreement delineating the program of one-to-one assistance that Anthony was receiving, that the district would maintain the assistance at the current level, and the level of support that the program and behavior specialists would continue to provide. We agreed to have a telephone conference in a month and a half to review the effectiveness of the program. If the program continued to be effective for Anthony, we then would sign a final mediation agreement, which is what occurred.

Observation and Another IEP Meeting

I went to observe Anthony in Ms. De Champ's class about a month after our IEP meeting. When I arrived, I was able to briefly see Anthony on the playground playing softball. When he returned to the classroom, a student peer tutor was with him for about thirty minutes. Ms. De Champ presented two short lessons to the entire class with a lot of student interaction and then broke the class up into smaller groups of three and four students. The lessons were all language-based, such as reading and repeating color words from the chalkboard, giving the sound of certain vowels (for example, short "a" sound) and consonants, and then sounding out consonant-vowel-consonant words that included those vowels and consonants. Anthony was able to read all the words of the colors correctly. He could sound out the vowels and consonants but was unable to put them together to make words. Another small group activity involved the students following one-step verbal directions (e.g., "Put an X on the bear." "Draw a circle around the fish.")

Anthony was on task for a good portion of the time, although he was easily distracted. He was able to read all the color words on the chalkboard. He knew the sounds of certain consonants (e.g., b, s, and m) and the short "a" sound, but had trouble sounding out consonant-vowel-consonant words. He could follow one-step directions, but had trouble somewhat with two-step directions. I was pleased to see that Ms. De Champ had incorporated more small-group instruction into her classroom activities than she had previously. It seemed to me that the program and behavior specialists' observations and consultation were positively influencing her teaching.

Several weeks later, toward the end of May, there was another IEP meeting for Anthony. This meeting was to review how he was progressing and talk about the program he would be in for the next school year. Ms. De Champ reported that Anthony had made significant progress and now was beginning to follow two-step directions. The behavior specialist reported on his working to reduce Anthony's hyperactive behavior when he entered the classroom. He also discussed how he was trying to prevent Anthony from becoming dependent on his student assistants. The school psychologist reported that Anthony answered her questions with two-word answers and she was trying to help him extend the length of his answers. We ended the meeting with my request to observe prospective class placements for Anthony for the following school year.

Moving with the Foster Family

Right before school let out for the summer, Angela contacted Pam to let her know that her family would be moving out of the county. Her husband had recently retired from the fire department and they wanted to move somewhere where the pace of life was slower and the community was safer. Angela wanted to find out what they would have to do so that Anthony could move with them sometime in the fall. Pam told her that she would talk with Nancy and they would determine what court procedures were required so that Anthony would be able to go with them.

When Pam shared the information with us that the Boltons would be moving and wanted to take Anthony with them; we were overjoyed that Anthony was considered an integral part of the Bolton family. We knew that he had received excellent care and support from the Boltons and he was thriving. We were sad, however, that our work on Anthony's behalf would be ending.

CONCLUSION

Angela Bolton became Anthony's guardian, which allowed Anthony to move with the family to their new home in another county. Anthony remained under the jurisdiction of the juvenile court in his county of origin at the urging of Nancy and Pam, which allowed the Boltons to continue receiving permanency placement services for Anthony from CPS.

The successful outcome of Anthony's case was primarily due to the fact that after a difficult early life and a grossly inappropriate placement once he entered foster care, he finally ended up in a foster family where he became a member of a well-functioning family. He was well cared for, had appropriate limits set for him, and was appreciated. Nevertheless, without the advocacy that took place by Advocacy Services, Anthony might never have landed with a foster family; and, once placed there, the foster family placement likely would have unraveled.

Nancy worked diligently, and with a clear vision, to have Anthony removed from the inappropriate group home placement. Once Anthony was placed with the Boltons, this placement might have been jeopardized if Angela Bolton had to continue picking up Anthony from school, sometimes on a daily basis, because of his behavior. This school placement was clearly not right for him, but his foster mother was not able to make any headway in bringing about a school placement change by herself.

Once Anthony was moved to a class for children with language disorders, and particularly after he started taking medication for his hyperactivity during the school day, he began progressing both academically and socially. Working with the school district through the special education mediation process was hugely instrumental in improving the class placement for him. The teacher's skills improved and Anthony had assistance to help him maintain attention and focus on instruction. Finally, Advocacy Services was able to help Anthony's foster mother become his legal guardian, enabling the family to take him with them when they moved to a new home in another county. Anthony, having become a true member of his foster family, flourished.

SUMMARY

The purpose of this chapter was to illuminate how inaccurate assessment information can result in a grossly inappropriate placement for a foster child with special needs. The chapter also highlighted how even when a child is placed in a nurturing foster family that an inappropriate school placement, where the foster parent has to be available to take the child home from school on a moment's notice for problem behavior, has the very real potential of jeopardizing the home placement. The chapter further explicated how an advocate for the child can work with the school district, through the special education appeal procedures, to strengthen a school program so that it adequately meets the needs of the child.

Chapter 11

David:
Working with a Court-Appointed
Special Advocate
to Reunite Separated Siblings

INTRODUCTION

David's case raises several important issues that have not yet been
encountered in the other cases in this book. These issues focus on the
adoption of foster youths and, in David's case, adoptions that are not
consummated. When should parental rights of a foster child's birth
parents be terminated? What are the consequences of terminating
parental rights of birth parents if a child is not adopted? What is the
legal relationship of siblings when the parental rights of their birth
parents are terminated? In addition to these questions, this chapter
also looks at the efforts of David's court-appointed special advocate
(CASA) and attorney to reunite him with his brother and try to address
his desperate need for nurturing and stability.

David, a white male, was removed, at seventeen months, from
his substance-abusing mother because of her neglect of him and his
brother. His parents' parental rights were terminated and he spent
seven years in the home of a foster parent whom he considered his
mother. When this foster mother felt that she no longer could care for
him because of his behavior, which she found disturbing, David com-
menced on a path of placement instability, hopping from one inappropriate placement to another, and always ending up in the county
emergency shelter.

The Systematic Mistreatment of Children in the Foster Care System
© 2007 by The Haworth Press, Taylor & Francis Group. All rights reserved.
doi:10.1300/5136_11

David's story demonstrates the widespread dysfunction for any child when his need for placement stability and permanence are not achieved. The result for David was that he was out of school for long periods and his mental health seriously deteriorated over time.

CASE STUDY OF DAVID

David's mother had a history of drug abuse. David was exposed prenatally to drugs and suffered withdrawal symptoms from barbiturates at birth. CPS, however, did not remove David from his mother's care at this time.

Petition and Detention/Arraignment Hearing

Seventeen months later, CPS filed a petition with the juvenile court alleging that his mother had neglected him. The petition stated that David had no parent or guardian capable of caring for or supervising him. It described his mother as "under the influence" to such a degree as to be unable to care for her son.

Prevention

When CPS detained David, he was placed in a shelter foster home for his protection. At the arraignment hearing, the allegations of the petition were sustained and the court ordered that David be "suitably placed." David remained in the shelter foster home for three months and then CPS moved him to a foster home where he remained for seven years. He thought of his foster mother, Linda, as his mother (see Exhibit 11.1).

Adoption Planning

David's social worker, when he was four-and-a-half, thought he was adoptable and, therefore, referred his case to the CPS Adoption Unit. His father's whereabouts had been unknown since David's birth. He had never made any inquiries to try to find his son. So when David was five, the juvenile court, at the request of CPS, terminated

EXHIBIT 11.1.
Placement History

Child's Age	Placement	Maltreatment	School
17 mos.	Shelter foster home	Neglect	Not in school
2 yrs.	Foster home		Not in school
6 yrs. 9 mos.	Foster home		Granite Elem.
8 yrs. 9 mos.	Kingman Group Home		Millbrook Elem.
10 yrs. 7 mos.	Kingman Group Home		Lucerne Elem.
10 yrs. 10 mos.	Emergency Shelter		Shelter School
10 yrs. 11 1/2 mos.	Foster Home		Home teacher
11 yrs. 1 mo.	Fulton Group Home		M.H. Clinic School
11 yrs. 3 mos.	Emergency Shelter		Shelter School
11 yrs. 4 mos.	Foster Home		Not in school
11 yrs. 6 mos.	Emergency Shelter		Shelter School
11 yrs 7 mos.	Group Home		Elem. School
11 yrs. 8 mos.	Emergency Shelter		Shelter School
12 yrs.	Pine Grove Residential		Pine Grove NPS
13 yrs. 3 mos.	Foster Home		Ashmore School

Elem. = Elementary School.

M.H. = Mental Health.

NPS = Nonpublic School (i.e., a private special education school).

his father's rights as David's parent. CPS argued that David's father effectively had abandoned his son.

A year later, CPS requested that David's mother voluntarily relinquish her parental rights to David, which she did. She believed David would be adopted.

David's legal status after the termination of his parents' rights was as a *legally freed minor*. His birth parents no longer were considered his parents. What David did not know, at this time, was that he had a half brother, Raymond, who was a year and five months younger than he was. The brothers both had been removed from the mother's custody and care at the same time. However, CPS never placed the boys together in the same foster home or even let them know that the other existed. When the court terminated their father and mother's parental rights to David, it also terminated their parental rights to Raymond. So Raymond also was considered a legally freed minor. As a result, David and Raymond legally were no longer considered brothers. Unfortunately, neither the adoption of David nor Raymond came to fruition, which led the court to order CPS to provide permanent foster care placement services for them.

What Had Gone Wrong?

CPS failed to ensure that David and Raymond were able to maintain and build their relationship even though they had been removed from the custody of their mother and ultimately her parental rights were terminated. The attorney who represented the boys should have made sure that procedures were securely in place for the brothers to continue a relationship with each other.

Advocacy Considerations

Current recommended practice for adoption is to terminate parental rights at the same court hearing that an adoption becomes legal. The Adoption and Safe Families Act (AFSA) associates the termination of parental rights with adoption. However, a judge could order continued sibling contact for biological half brothers, such as David and Raymond (see Exhibit 11.2).

Some states have enacted laws addressing sibling rights (Schweitzer & Larson, 2005). One such law states: "Any siblings who are separated

EXHIBIT 11.2.
Adoption and Safe Families Act

The Adoption and Safe Families Act (1997) requires that termination of parental rights proceedings be initiated for children who have been under the responsibility of the state for fifteen out of the most recent twenty-two months that they have been in foster care. The state agency, concurrently with its filing of a termination of parental rights petition, must identify, recruit, process, and approve a qualified family for adoption. The exceptions to initiating the termination of parental rights proceedings are: (1) the child is in the care of a relative; (2) the state agency documents a compelling reason why filing is not in the best interest of the child; or (3) the state agency has not provided to the child's family, consistent with the time period in the case plan, the services deemed necessary to return the child to a safe home.

due to a foster care or adoptive placement may petition a court, including a juvenile court with jurisdiction over one or more of the siblings, for reasonable sibling visitation rights" (*Sibling Placement and Visitation Rights,* 2006, §5-525.2b).

The federal department of health and human services currently conducts Child and Family Services Reviews (CFSR)—comprehensive assessments of state child welfare programs—under Title IV-B and Title IV-E of the Social Security Act. One of the permanency outcome measures under which states are evaluated is preserving continuity of family relationships. Two of the categories considered under this outcome measure are placement of children with siblings and preserving connections with family.

Problems Surface

David's foster mother, Linda, did not send him to preschool. When he began formal schooling, difficulty with self-control surfaced early. In kindergarten, he exhibited problems controlling his behavior and working independently. His kindergarten teacher wrote in his school cumulative file "needs help in self-control, average achievement academically."

David was evaluated in the first grade to determine whether he qualified for special education services, but was found ineligible because he did not have a specific learning disability, according to his individualized education program (IEP) team. His IEP states: "It appears that his behavior problems in the classroom are a deterrent to his learning. He appears to be functioning age-appropriately with no signs of learning disabilities at this time." The IEP team recommended that the classroom teacher use a behavior modification program to improve David's behavior. Even though David did not qualify for special education services, the school still provided him with some counseling services. David's first grade teacher wrote in his cumulative file: "[David] had some difficulty relating. He does not complete work independently. [He is] improving in reading with the help from reading lab but still below grade level. He has limited self-confidence. [David] participated in the counseling group with the school psychologist and . . . has shown improvement."

A year later, when David was in second grade and his problem behavior continued, his social worker referred him for another evaluation for special education. This time, however, based on the testing and classroom observations, David was found to have a specific learning disability and, therefore, was found eligible for special education services.

At the end of the school year, David's second grade teacher wrote the following comments in his cumulative file: "[David] has been getting help from our Resource Lab and it has been helping. His behavior has improved over last year. He is beginning to take more responsibility for his actions. His math skills are on grade level. He needs lots of individual help in reading to keep him on task."

What Had Gone Wrong?

Why is it that in the first grade, David was not found to have a specific learning disability, but in the second grade, he was and, on that basis, became eligible for special education services? David's scores on standardized tests he took when he was in the first grade, were, except for one subtest score in math, all at the first grade level. In addition, his IEP team attributed whatever academic problems

David was having in class at this time to his problem behavior. So the team did not conclude that he had a specific learning disability.

By the second grade, David's standardized test scores in reading, spelling, and general information were still at the first grade level. The psychologist evaluating him now gave him some additional tests to assess his perceptual motor skills, his memory, his ability to learn, and his self-concept. With this more comprehensive assessment and the fact that he was a year older made his skill deficits show the requisite discrepancy from his assumed average intelligence. In the psychologist's report, she also indicated that she observed behavior from David that was indicative of serious emotional problems. His IEP indicates that he has an "emotional overlay," yet there were no goals, objectives, or services to address the emotional/behavioral issues (see Exhibit 11.3).

Change in Foster Home Placement

David's behavior problems at the foster home became increasingly more difficult for Linda to handle. Linda also reported that David destroyed property; he would tear clothing and break toys and furniture. He engaged in fights where he would hit and kick other children who lived in the home. She found David either withdrawn or angry and destructive. In addition, according to Linda, David continued to wet his bed and engaged in excessive masturbation. It was the excessive masturbation that finally drove her to request that the social worker find David another home.

So, when David was eight years and nine months, in the middle of his third grade year, his social worker moved him to the Kingman

---

EXHIBIT 11.3.
Specific Learning Disability

The 2004 reauthorization of the Individuals with Disabilities Education Act allows school districts to change the way they determine whether a child has a specific learning disability. The new eligibility criteria do not require a discrepancy between ability and achievement, but rather look at a child's response to intervention. (IDEA, 2004)

Group Home, where Martha Kingman was the owner. The change in placement required that he change schools. Since Linda's foster home was the only home David had known, and he thought of her as his mother, this was a most difficult time for him. Prior to changing schools, David's third grade teacher at his school wrote in his cumulative file: "[David] still attends Resource Lab. He can do his math skills reasonably well. He has a short attention span and needs individual help constantly."

A Court-Appointed Special Advocate Assigned

A court-appointed special advocate (CASA) named Richard Johnston was assigned to David and his brother. His initial charge was to explore how the boys were faring and whether sibling visits would be in their best interests.

At the court hearing, shortly after CPS placed David in the Kingman Group Home, Richard reported to the judge that David did not want to stay at the group home. He desperately wanted to return to Linda's home and complained that he did not like the other boys in the Kingman home. The CASA told the judge that Martha Kingman had reported that David was a very disturbed boy. She said that one of the staff members who worked at the home told her that David had a self-esteem problem and it would be helpful if something could be done to help him think better of himself. David's general education classroom teacher told the CASA that she had serious concerns' about David's lack of progress academically and his aggressive behavior. Based on all of this information, the judge ordered psychological counseling for David and Raymond and that the boys were to receive psychological evaluations. He also ordered CPS to facilitate visits between the brothers.

Psychological Evaluation

Based on the court order, CPS referred David to a psychologist who evaluated him to determine his current functioning level and to assist in program planning and placement. The psychologist interviewed David, gave him an IQ test, a test of perceptual motor ability, and several projective tests. In her report, the psychologist described David's affect as bland and subdued, exhibiting little range of emotion. He was withdrawn and spoke in a soft, at times, inaudible voice. He was compliant with her requests of him and interacted in a polite appropriate fashion. Although she felt he displayed reasonable effort during the evaluation, she found him to be depressed and felt he suffered from a poorly identified self-concept and low self-esteem. She also saw him as desirous of closeness, but fearful of the intimacy so he typically acted in ways to keep others distant from him. Her diagnostic impression was that David had dysthymia (i.e., depression), attention deficit disorder, and borderline intellectual functioning. She found that his fund of relevant facts about the world was highly restricted, but felt that his borderline intellectual functioning might be an underestimation of his true ability due to his distractibility and impulsivity.

The psychologist recommended that David receive a neuropsychological examination to identify the possible existence of organic impairment thus limiting his intellectual, emotional, and social functioning. She felt that the evaluation results supported placement of David in a special education classroom. In addition, because he lacked exposure to consistent, positive, nurturing role models, she recommended that he be referred for a "Big Brother."

What Had Gone Wrong?

The psychologist correctly concluded that David's IQ score was likely to be an underestimation of his ability due to his distractibility and impulsivity. There is reason to suspect, for this population of children, that the scores that place them in the borderline intellectual functioning range frequently are an underestimation of their ability. Part of the concern is that the tests used have not specifically been "normed" on foster youths, so it may be unclear what the scores actually mean for this population of students. In David's case, there are additional reasons to be wary of the results of his intelligence testing because of his depressed state at the time and his distractibility and impulsivity.

Neuropsychological Evaluation

Two months later, based on the recommendation of the psychologist who had evaluated David, he was given a neuropsychological evaluation. This evaluator found that nearly all functional areas tested showed some signs of deficiency or impairment. There were signs of significant impairment on tasks of abstract reasoning and concept formation, verbal fluency, verbal comprehension, reading, spelling, arithmetic, auditory and visual memory, and attention and concentration. Intact areas were tactile and visual sensory perception as well as motor functioning.

Based on the results of this evaluation, the psychologist recommended that David should be placed in a full-day special education program because he did not have the intellectual or the emotional resources to function adequately in a regular classroom setting. He felt that David was in need of specialized forms of academic instruction due to his generalized cognitive dysfunction. This instruction should be provided in a small, supervised learning environment with direct teacher supervision to help reduce the disruptive effects of his emotional disturbance on learning. This setting also would provide greater control over competing and distracting stimuli than a regular classroom setting as well as provide a greater amount of individualized attention.

Advocacy Considerations

There has been an ongoing, often heated, debate in the special education community on the issue of full inclusion for all special education students on general education school campuses and in general education classrooms (Kavale & Forness, 2000). Those who endorse full inclusion would argue that David could have been maintained in a general education class if proper supports had been brought to the classroom. Others, who do not hold this perspective, would likely agree with the psychologist who did the neuropsychological evaluation that David needed a small structured environment that could only be achieved in a full-day special education class (see Exhibit 11.4).

Special Day Class Placement

Martha Kingman shared the recently completed psychological evaluation with the psychologist from David's school and requested that his special education placement be changed from the part-time resource specialist program to a full-day special day class. The school psychologist did her own psychoeducational evaluation of David.

EXHIBIT 11.4.
Least Restrictive Environment and Full Inclusion

The IDEA requires that students with disabilities are educated and participate with students without disabilities to the maximum extent appropriate. The Courts of Appeal in *Daniel R.R. v. El Paso Independent School District* (1989), *Greer v. Rome City School District* (1991), *Board of Education v. Holland* (1994) and *Ronker v. Walter* (1983) make it clear that the decision to remove a child with a disability from the general education classroom or school is not one to be taken lightly. A major effort must be taken, by supplementing the general education environment with aids and services, to make that environment appropriate for the child with a disability.

A month later, toward the end of the summer, the school district scheduled an IEP meeting to review the school psychologist's findings and to make a determination about his special education program for the new school year. David recently had turned nine and was about to start the fourth grade. His third grade teacher from Millbrook Elementary wrote the following comments in David's cumulative file at the end of the third grade: "[David] is weak in all social and academic areas. He needs to feel that he is loved. He is a very angry child."

The school psychologist concluded, based on measures of adaptive behavior, work samples, achievement tests, school records, teacher input, observations, and professional judgment, that David's overall cognitive ability was low average, although there were some areas where he performed somewhat higher. Academically, he was significantly behind in all areas and was functioning, based on standardized assessment instruments, at about the middle of the first grade level. He was able to add and subtract two and three column numbers requiring simple regrouping, but he could not multiply or divide. He had no real phonetic approach to reading and had poor common sight word recognition. He had trouble printing all the letters of the alphabet. On a behavior rating scale, he received a "very significant" score in the areas of poor attention, academics, impulse control, sense of identity, anger control, ego strength, and coordination. His ratings were in the "significant" range in the areas of excessive resistance, aggressiveness, and withdrawal. Additional testing showed problems in David's receptive language and his ability to do visual perceptual motor tasks. He was above average on tasks requiring auditory discrimination. David's eligibility based on a specific learning disability continued, but the IEP team recommended a placement change to a special day class for students with learning disabilities and counseling for thirty minutes per week by the school psychologist.

IEP Meeting

Five months after the previous IEP meeting, David's CPS social worker requested a review IEP meeting to determine whether David would be better served in a special day class for students with serious emotional disturbance, rather than the one he had been in for students with learning disabilities. This IEP described David as respecting adult authority, but having poor peer relationships and lacking impulse control. He had delays in expressive language and, although he was able to verbally express his needs, he had not learned to use verbal language to deal with problem situations but instead used aggression. The IEP team decided to make David's primary category for special education eligibility emotional disturbance, because his behavior at school had deteriorated in recent months. The team also recommended placement in a special day class for students with this disability, which meant that David had to change schools since Millbrook did not have this type of classroom program. Consequently, David started attending Lucerne Elementary, which was farther from his home and required a longer bus ride.

Court Review Hearing

At a six-month juvenile court review hearing, held a month after his IEP meeting, David's social worker reported that he demonstrated disruptive behaviors at home and at school. He reported that the police had picked David up on at least one occasion for shoplifting, but no charges were filed. He also indicated that David frequently ran away from home and school. The social worker reported that David recently had an IEP meeting and he now was receiving his special education services in a class for students with serious emotional disturbances.

David's CASA described him in a more positive light. The CASA reported that David now liked where he was living and appeared to be better adjusted to the Kingman Group Home. He attributed this change to Martha Kingman having hired a new staff person for the home who was able to spend more individual time with him and keep his behavior problems under control.

What Had Gone Wrong?

What neither David's CPS social worker nor CASA shared with the court was that David desperately wanted to visit with his former foster mother, Linda. He clearly missed not being with her. However, for visits to occur, David's social worker had to approve them and make arrangements, such as scheduling and transportation. The social worker had decided that it was not a good idea for David to see his former foster mother, because he attributed David's deteriorating behavior to times when he did see Linda. So the social worker did not do anything to bring about future visits. Consequently, David ran away on a consistent basis from both the group home and school and always ended up at his former foster home. The group home staff punished David for running away, rather than understanding his emotional need to see Linda.

David was not yet ten at this time, and had to travel quite a distance through gang-ridden urban neighborhoods to reach Linda's home. Clearly, such travel posed a serious risk of harm to David. During this time, David's behavior at school deteriorated significantly leading to the IEP meeting where he was identified as having an emotional disturbance and placed in a classroom with other students with this disability. It is easy to see how David's anger and depression about his home life negatively affected his ability to function at school.

Appointment of Advocacy Services and Change in CASA

At the end of the summer, when David was ten years and two months, the juvenile court appointed Nancy to represent both David and his brother Raymond. At about the same time, Richard Johnston, David's CASA, was not able to continue on David and Raymond's case. So, Diana Gorsky, whose children were grown leaving her time to devote to volunteer activities, was appointed as the new CASA.

IEP Meeting

Soon after Diana was appointed as David's CASA, there was an IEP meeting held, which she attended. David now was halfway through his fifth grade year in the special day class at Lucerne Elementary. At the meeting, David's teacher reported he was able to read material at the second grade level with great difficulty. He substituted some consonant sounds and omitted others so his oral reading was not fluent and his independent work was minimal. At the same time, he was able to add and subtract with regrouping in the tens and hundreds places and was beginning to learn multiplication facts and concepts. Poor study skills and follow through were conditions that hampered his progress in spelling and writing. His dysfunctional behaviors in class included teasing peers, confronting them in a combative stance, and being noncompliant with adults. Noted on this IEP was that David had left the school site without permission. The recommendation emanating from this meeting was for David to continue in the special day class for students with serious emotional disturbance and to receive counseling from the school psychologist for thirty minutes per week. The group-home owner signed the IEP as David's parent.

What Had Gone Wrong?

First of all, the group-home owner should not have signed David's IEP as his parent. Instead, Diana Gorsky, the CASA, should have been appointed as his surrogate parent to sign the IEP and thus authorize his special education services. Federal and state special education law requires that a child who does not have a parent be appointed a surrogate parent. The law requires that a surrogate parent not have any interests that conflict with the child's interests and not be an employee of the state. Group-home owners are considered to have a possible conflict of interest with the children's needs since group homes are considered businesses. The owners or staff, therefore, might not always advocate for the child's needs if those needs required additional time, say, to transport the child to a different school or if they led to a different home placement.

Disagreement Between CPS and the CASA

When Diana Gorsky was appointed as David's CASA, one of the first things she did was to visit him at his group home. She was appalled at the condition of the Kingman Group Home. There was hardly any furniture in the house (although there was a broken television set), and there were no toys at all with which the children could play. Diana also was quite upset about David continuing to be punished for running away to Linda's house. She learned, during one of her visits, that David was extremely upset because he and the other boys in the home were not able to participate in a Boys' and Girls' Club Basketball League because the group-home owner said she had no extra staff to transport the children to the practices or the games.

Diana contacted David's social worker to try to arrange for David to have visits with his former foster mother and to attempt to bring about a change of placement for him. The social worker, having originally approved the placement for David, was resistant to make a change now. In fact, he not only was resistant to the CASA's suggestions, he also wrote a letter to the director of the CASA office and to the juvenile court judge criticizing Diana for unprofessional behavior related to her work on David's case. This letter was in response to Diana's report to the court that pointed out areas where the social worker had not followed through on a variety of matters related to David. Diana also reported on how Linda had been trying from the time that David was placed in the Kingman Group Home to arrange for him to visit her. She told the judge how upset David was about this and the vague reasons the social worker had given for not allowing the visits.

What Had Gone Wrong?

CASAs can play an important role both in spending extended time with a child to try to understand the child's needs and in providing in-depth information to the court, relevant to the child's case. However, tension between a CASA and the other people in the child's life sometimes erupts, particularly when caregivers do not like having another person "looking over their shoulders" and reporting problems they find to the court. In David's case, the social worker did not like the CASA questioning his judgment and criticizing his actions, so he fought back by providing a critical report of the CASA to the court. Obviously, it is better for the child if this tension does not exist since CASAs and social workers should be working together in mutually supportive roles to further the best interests of the child. When conflicting information is presented to the court, the judge has to determine whose position he finds most credible.

Further Concern About the Group Home

Nancy decided to visit David in the group home to see the conditions for herself. She too was appalled at the inadequate conditions of the home. While she was there, she talked to the staff about not punishing David for running away to his previous foster home. Shortly after Nancy's visit, David ran away again. When CPS picked him up, he pleaded not to be sent back to the group home and alleged that he was being physically abused there. This time, David need not have worried about going back to the Kingman Group Home for the group-home owner had refused to take him back.

Emergency Shelter

David remained at the emergency shelter for about a month and a half. While he was there, he earned more points than did any of the other boys on his living unit for good behavior, thus enabling him to move to an honor dormitory.

While at the emergency shelter, David received a psychiatric evaluation and medication monitoring by a psychiatric team from a local university hospital. At the time, he had been taking Mellaril (a tranquilizer and low potency antipsychotic drug often used to treat behavior problems in children) for two years. The psychiatrist gradually lowered the dosage of Mellaril, since David's behavior was fine, and then took him off the medication totally. David did extremely well while off Mellaril, so the doctor's report stated that no medication was warranted at that time. He also reported that David did not meet the criteria for attention deficit hyperactivity disorder.

While at the emergency shelter, the student planning team referred David for a language screening because he appeared to have difficulty expressing his thoughts. After failing the screening, he was given an in-depth language assessment. The results of assessment were that

David demonstrated a significant language disorder characterized by deficits in grammatical and syntactical constructions and receptive and expressive semantic skills. He had difficulty in identifying correct words for items, putting words into categories, interpreting critical concepts and word meanings in sentences, and providing meanings for synonyms and antonyms. The speech and language specialist found that his language lacked the flexibility and specificity of children his age. He also had difficulty in correctly formulating compound and complex sentences with conjunctions.

Another IEP meeting was held where, in addition to the services he was to receive from the resource specialist, psychologist, and a behavior management assistant, speech and language services were added to his IEP. At the IEP meeting, his CASA reported that he had left his previous school district before the referral to DMH had been completed. But the IEP team did not initiate another referral.

What Had Gone Wrong?

The fact that David did so well at the emergency shelter seems to indicate that the previous settings he was in were not appropriate for him or, perhaps, not appropriate for any child. Furthermore, his removal from Mellaril and ability to behave appropriately also indicate that the Kingman Group Home placement had been an emotional disaster for him.

In relation to the determination that he had a language disorder, David clearly should have been referred previously for an assessment of his language skills. For youth with emotional and behavioral problems, however, sometimes their behavior often obscures other learning problems that they have.

Psychological Assessment

Around the time David entered the emergency shelter, CPS assigned him a new social worker, Bob Sheffield. One of the first things that Bob did was to report David's allegation of physical abuse (i.e., being hit by staff) at the Kingman Group Home to the state department of social services. He then referred David for a psychological evaluation to help determine a suitable placement for him.

The psychologist who evaluated David described him in her report as generally cooperative and interacting appropriately during the evaluation, but he was seemingly sad. There were no signs of behavioral acting out. David's score on an IQ test was in the borderline range of intellectual functioning, but his pattern of subtest scores suggested uneven cognitive development, with some scores in the average range. The psychologist suggested that it was highly probable that David had not been exposed to a wide variety of educational experiences. Subtests, which required skills that were dependent on academic achievement showed serious deficits. His average scores were on subtests assessing ability to read environmental and situational cues and from these cues make appropriate decisions and judgments. The psychologist cautioned, however, that David's decision-making skills might not be adequate if he were in a highly emotional state.

On a test of visual motor functioning, David was unable to copy designs from cards with any degree of accuracy. In some cases, he was unable even to come close to reproducing the designs. The psychologist reported that the data from this test clearly reflected a significant perceptual motor impairment.

From the projective tests given, the psychologist found that David experienced himself as powerless and insignificant. The themes from these tests were of sadness, abandonment, physical fragility, and violent attack. She felt he was quite a sad and depressed boy, who had thought of giving up on life due to recent losses and the lack of stability in his life. There was evidence of suicidal ideation, but not current evidence of David intending or planning to harm himself.

The psychologist recommended that David be placed in a small, specialized foster home that could meet some of his needs for a family and, ideally, that he could reunify with his former foster mother, Linda. She also recommended that David receive psychological counseling to work on issues of loss and self-esteem and that he be referred for a medication consultation for antidepressants. She wanted him monitored for suicidal ideation since he showed a significant amount of depression and a strong sense of hopelessness. She felt it would help him if a schedule were established for maintaining contact with significant others in his life, such as his former foster mother and foster children he had lived with in her home. He also needed a referral to an optician for glasses, having been examined earlier in the year but not having received glasses.

Foster Home Placement

CPS next placed David in a foster home with one other boy there. David was now ten years and eleven months. The social worker, who made the placement, Victor Drummond, recently had been assigned to David's case, since Bob Sheffield now was moved to another CPS office in the county. David only lasted in this foster home a little over a month before he ended up back at the emergency shelter. Part of the problem of this placement was that the foster father was unable to enroll David in school. The school district claimed it could not enroll David until it received his previous IEPs and other education records. After receiving these documents, the district then wanted to assess David before placing him in a classroom. During this time, the district provided David with twenty minutes of daily instruction by a home teacher. Since the foster father worked long hours out of the home, not having David in school was a real problem. The foster father's mother was at home during the day, but she and David did not get along very well.

It took almost a month to get David into school. His CASA intervened and tracked down the school records that the district wanted. David eventually was placed in one of the district's special education classes for students with serious emotional disturbance. Soon after, David ran away from his foster home one night when the foster father was gone. When the police picked David up, he told them he wanted to go to the emergency shelter.

What Had Gone Wrong?

Clearly, the school district holding up David's enrollment in school helped to jeopardize this foster home placement. The district should have immediately enrolled David in school. Having a current IEP from the emergency shelter school should have been sufficient. Because many foster children spend an enormous amount of time out of school when they change home placements, particularly those children who receive special education services, the state where David lived passed legislation (AB 490, 2003) requiring school districts to immediately enroll foster youths in school, even if they come without school or immunization records. This legislation will be discussed further in Chapter 12.

Brothers Placed in Group Home Together

David's brother Raymond had been living in the same foster home for five years when CPS became aware that his foster mother did not have a proper license from the state. Consequently, all of the boys in the home were removed. At the same time, beds become available at a recently opened group home for boys with emotional problems between the ages of nine and twelve. So, with the urging of their CASA, David and Raymond both were placed at the Fulton Group Home. Diana had been taking the boys on outings so they could get to know each other and they both were enjoying their time together.

Victor Drummond took David and Raymond to the Fulton Group Home in the middle of the summer. Not too long after their placement there, Nancy contacted the group-home owner, Elizabeth Fulton, and learned that David and Raymond were not getting along and their behavior problems were escalating. She also learned that both boys now were taking Mellaril.

Diana's initial visit to the home, when the boys were first placed there, was positive. At that first meeting, she liked Elizabeth Fulton, the group-home owner.

This time, however, when she went to visit David and Raymond, she became concerned about their well-being. What she observed was David's constant tormenting and beating up his younger brother. Diana suggested to the group-home owner that the boys might need some crisis counseling. Diana knew that Elizabeth did not take well to this suggestion, but was taken aback when she asked her not to visit the boys again. Elizabeth told her that her visits and calls were disruptive.

Diana was troubled by Elizabeth's request. She also was concerned that David and Raymond were together almost every minute of the day. They even were in the same class at the small school that was located on the grounds of a nearby mental health clinic. The class only had a few other students, all of whom had serious mental health disorders.

Nancy went to visit the Fulton Group Home and found David extremely angry. He told her again and again that he was going to run away to Linda's home and that he wanted to live with Linda and that just visiting her would not be enough. He also confided to Nancy that he really did not want to leave Raymond. Raymond, on the other hand, told Nancy that he hated David and did not want to live with him. By the end of the meeting, both boys had somewhat settled down.

It became evident to Nancy that the Fulton Group Home was not right for David or Raymond. She was uncomfortable with the way Elizabeth Fulton was handling the problems between the boys and that she had prohibited Diana from seeing them. She also was concerned because neither of the boys wanted to stay there and seemed almost despondent about their current living situation. Nancy talked with the social worker about her concerns. After talking with his supervisor, he told Nancy that the boys would remain at the Fulton Group Home.

Nancy then decided she would have to obtain a court order if she wanted the boys out of the group home. So, with Diana's help and the help of Marianne Obani, supervisor of the CASA program, she was prepared to ask the court to order the removal of David and Raymond from the Fulton Group Home. However, when Nancy went into court to request the court order, she learned that CPS was opposing her request. The lawyer representing CPS argued strongly for not granting the order to remove the boys from the Fulton Group Home. He argued that the group home provided a good treatment setting with appropriate care and intervention. Marianne Obani, the CASA program supervisor, on the other hand, discussed their extreme unhappiness with their current living situation, documented by their CASA, Diana Gorsky. David and Raymond also had complained that their arms hurt from constantly being physically restrained by group-home staff. Elizabeth Fulton had told Diana that it was necessary to physically restrain the boys when they acted out.

The CASA program supervisor relayed how the psychologist at their school said that David and Raymond were not functioning well and seemed to have lost all motivation. He told her that the other children placed in the Fulton Home had not done well emotionally and he had misgivings about the treatment they received. Their teacher said that Raymond spent the entire day sucking his thumb and that without intensive intervention "he'd be lost." The CASA supervisor also reported how Elizabeth Fulton would not let Diana see the boys and had refused to take any phone calls from her, or to let David or Raymond even speak to her. Elizabeth Fulton reportedly told Diana that she would fight to the end to keep the boys and prevent any interference from her or anyone else from the CASA program. After hearing the concerns about the group home raised by the CASA supervisor, the judge ordered David and Raymond removed from the Fulton Group Home (see Exhibit 11.5).

What Had Gone Wrong?

Elizabeth Fulton did not like the CASA's involvement in David and Raymond's lives. She did not like someone "meddling" in how she ran her group home. This led her to attempt to ban Diana from seeing or talking to David and Raymond. She did not seem to understand the role of a CASA. Diana had been appointed by the court explicitly to keep the judge informed about the needs of the children. In addition, both boys were feeling deep losses from having been removed from foster homes where they had lived for many years and had bonded with their foster mothers. Since they each had a connection with Diana, it was important that she continue to be a steady presence in their lives.

The fact that David and Raymond were physically restrained at Elizabeth Fulton's group home on a regular basis was a clear indication that something was wrong. The boys needed skilled, nurturing caretakers who could set appropriate limits for them, but also could make them feel cared about and empathize with their feelings of loss.

Diana, although good intentioned, seems to have been somewhat unrealistic in assuming that putting David and Raymond together in the same home would improve their lives automatically. However, she could not have known that the treatment the boys would receive

EXHIBIT 11.5.
The Role of Court-Appointed Special Advocates

Court-appointed special advocates (CASAs) play an important role in informing the juvenile court about the needs of foster children and recommending placements and services.

in this home would be so detrimental to their well-being. Nancy, too, had gone along with the plan of placing them together with the hope that it would work out well.

Most horrifying, however, was that CPS was protecting this group-home owner. Nancy learned that senior level administrators at CPS had instructed their attorney to fight Nancy's request for a court order to remove the boys from the group home because Elizabeth Fulton had "friends in high places." It was never clear who these "friends" were.

To his credit, the judge did not let CPS or its lawyer intimidate him. He took quite seriously the reports written by David and Raymond's CASA and her supervisor detailing the failings of the Fulton Group Home placement and the recommendation to remove them from that setting. The CASA supervisor, contrary to her usual practice, came to the court herself to present her report. The judge ultimately appears to have been swayed by the CASA's reports and the strong conviction of the supervisor that removal of the boys from this placement was absolutely necessary.

Continual Return to the Emergency Shelter

David and Raymond were placed in the emergency shelter. This change of placement occurred only a little over two months after David and Raymond had first been placed at the Fulton Group Home. Shortly after their return to the emergency shelter, a bed became available at a very well thought of residential treatment facility. Raymond was placed there, where he did quite well. David stayed at the emergency shelter for another month and then was placed in another foster home, where he lasted less than two months. He was defiant with the foster mother, stole money from her, refused to go to school, and ultimately ran away when she yelled at him and was returned to the emergency shelter. This time, after three weeks at the emergency shelter, CPS placed him in the Castle Group Home, where he lasted about a month and a half before engaging in such destructive behavior that the police were called and brought him to the emergency shelter.

Request for a Stopgap Placement

In order to try to stop the vicious placement and replacement cycle that David seemed to be caught in, Nancy requested that David's social worker have him screened for the special program that CPS had instituted for hard-to-place youngsters. This was the same program that Sharon was in, the Stopgap program. It was a program where the county gave a residential treatment facility substantially more money per month for the child, in return for the facility agreeing not to discharge the youngster. In effect, it was a bonus for taking on difficult cases.

At the next court hearing, Diana reported to the court on David's recent placement history. She described how he had failed five group home or foster home placements in the last ten months and made a case for his need for a residential treatment program. She specifically requested that he become a part of the Stopgap program. Diana stated that it was time for David to stop this destructive pattern of deliberately failing placements and being returned to the emergency shelter. She informed the judge that David had hardly attended school in the last ten months because of constantly changing home placements. She also expressed concern that at every foster or group home placement he had been in the last ten months, he was put on medication (i.e., Mellaril) and then taken off of it when he returned to the emergency shelter. She noted that he always had done better while he was off Mellaril.

Stopgap Placement

While David was at the emergency shelter, he had been screened and accepted in the Stopgap Program. The residential treatment facility that accepted him was Pine Grove Residential.

Intervention

David had just turned twelve when he was placed at Pine Grove. He did quite well in the structured program. During his year and three months there, he started having visits with his former foster mother, Linda Hendricks. As his behavior improved, he was able to have overnight visits with her. Finally, Linda Hendricks decided to take David back into her home when he was discharged from Pine Grove.

Placement with Former Foster Mother

When David was thirteen years and three months, he moved back into Linda Hendrick's home. This is what David had yearned for from the time, years before, when she felt she no longer could care for him. The staff at Pine Grove continued to provide aftercare services to David and Linda Hendricks to support the placement. He and his brother also started spending time together again.

CONCLUSION

David's case demonstrates how dire consequences can result from terminating parental rights and failing to attain permanency for a foster child. It also shows that reuniting siblings who never knew each other in the context of an inadequate group home setting will not necessarily erase their emotional and behavioral problems nor substitute for the permanent parental relationship for which they both longed.

David's case shows how important it is to support, with intensive wraparound services if necessary, the placement of a child with a long-term foster parent even when problems arise that can cause the foster parent to feel that the arrangement is not working. David desperately wanted to be with this foster mother. What was particularly difficult for him was that, once removed from her home, the homes in which he was placed were absolutely inadequate in meeting his needs for nurturing, mental health treatment, and education. These were all places where his intense longing for visits with his former foster mother was ignored. The situation did not improve when David and his brother were placed in the same group home, because the home did not provide the kind of nurturing and support that he and his brother required and they both were suffering from the loss of long-term foster parents.

David's CASA worked tirelessly on his behalf and was successful against powerful stakeholders in having David removed from a group home that was deleterious to his well-being. But efforts to improve David's situation did not occur until he ultimately was reunited with the only person whom he could think of as his mother.

SUMMARY

The purpose of this chapter was to illuminate the problems that can arise when parental rights are terminated and children are not adopted. The chapter also shows the curious situation that can occur when biological brothers no longer have a legal relationship after the rights of their parents are terminated. For foster children who are not adopted, this chapter strongly makes clear how the problems they face are further exacerbated when they are removed from long-term foster home placements without the ability to maintain relationships with their former caretakers. This chapter also focuses on the role of a court-appointed special advocate (CASA) in the lives of foster children and the sometimes-difficult role that CASAs must play.

Chapter 12

Directions for Change

The cases of the children described in this book reveal enormous cracks in the systems of care, mental health, education, and other supports for children in foster care and their families. For foster youths with emotional and behavioral disorders, these cracks can be particularly deep and difficult to negotiate.

The cracks described in this book are not new and, in recent years, there have been important efforts to patch some of them. Nonetheless, there are still more changes that must occur, and those, which have been put into place, are not sufficiently effective to bring about permanency and well-being for many children like those described in this book.

The Adoption and Safe Families Act (AFSA), passed by the U.S. Congress in 1997, was an important step to begin dealing with the issue of permanency for youths in foster care. AFSA not only shortens timelines for putting children into permanent placements and provides incentives to improve adoption rates. It also requires accountability for child protective services (CPS) agencies to determine if their efforts are resulting in positive outcomes for foster youth.

Three years later, in 2000, the U.S. Department of Health and Human Services published a new review process, the Child and Family Services Review (CFSR), to evaluate state outcomes for children and families, and penalize states that are found out of compliance with these outcomes after giving them one to two years to correct the problems (Reed & Karpilow, 2002). The results of the recent CFSR process shows that states are especially weak in helping children achieve their permanency goals in a timely manner and in supporting families with services that they need to care for their children (Child Welfare League of America [CWLA], 2004).

The Systematic Mistreatment of Children in the Foster Care System
© 2007 by The Haworth Press, Taylor & Francis Group. All rights reserved.
doi:10.1300/5136_12

National reports by organizations such as the Child Welfare League of America (2004), the Annie E. Casey Foundation (Family to Family, 2001), and the Pew Charitable Trusts (Pew Commission on Children in Foster Care, 2004) also call attention to the growing number of children in out-of-home care and the steady decline in the pool of available foster families to provide temporary or permanent care. These reports express concern about a federal financing structure that encourages over-reliance on placement of children in foster care at the expense of other more permanent options for children.

Others have voiced their concerns about foster youths not attaining permanent stable homes. Courtney, Roderick, Smithgall, Gladden, and Nagoka (2004) write: "Despite increased efforts to reduce the amount of time that children spent in out-of-home placements, many of those who are in care spend considerable periods of time—often years—under the supervision of the child welfare system" (p. 1). Some have pointed out the failings of the foster care system in terms of not adequately serving foster youths.

> Foster youth not only have to cope with the trauma of separation from families unable or unwilling to provide proper care, but they also must live within a child protective system that is over-burdened and, in many cases, ill-equipped to provide even a basic level of stability, safety, and nurturing. (Youth Transition Funders Group, 2004, p. 6)

As the stories of the children in this book dramatically demonstrate, CPS, along with the other agencies, responsible for educating and providing mental health and other services to foster youth are part of a system that clearly does not work well for many of our most vulnerable children. Because the challenges of the children and their families are great, they typically require services from more than one agency. Unfortunately, the cracks within and between agencies frequently conspire to deny them essential services. These are children that the state has taken away from their parents because of parental substance abuse, mental illness, severe use of physical punishment, among other reasons, which have led to abuse or neglect. All too frequently, however, we put these children in out-of-home placements that are hardly better than the situations from which they were removed. We must do better for these children. We owe it to them.

This chapter looks closely at the fissures exposed in the multi-agency system of care by the advocates as they tried to attain, for the children described in this book, stable living environments, appropriate schooling, supportive mental health and other services that they desperately needed and, in most cases, to which they were entitled by law. What is essential is not only that the cracks be exposed, but also repaired so that other children who enter the foster care system will not fall so easily through them. Consequently, in addition to describing the categories of cracks that were found in the advocacy efforts, this chapter seeks to describe interventions and systemic policy changes that would help repair many of them. Some of the changes that are needed are already underway in various pilot projects across the country or have recently been put into law in individual states. Still, these piecemeal efforts, while significant, have not resulted in overall policy and program changes for many youths in foster care, particularly those with the greatest needs. Other necessary changes still must be realized.

CREATING STABLE HOME PLACEMENTS

One of the major cracks in the child welfare system that most of the children who are described in this book faced was that they could not be maintained in a stable living situation and were moved constantly from one out-of-home home placement to another. Patty had to endure eighteen different out-of-home placements, which, unfortunately, is not that exceptional for "difficult" children (see Exhibit 12.1).

EXHIBIT 12.1.
Placement Changes

The plight of children in the dependency system is sobering. In addition to dealing with the physical and emotional trauma of parental abuse or neglect, these children must struggle with numerous changes in their placement and their schools. In fact, foster children in California attend an average of nine to ten different schools by age eighteen. (Kelly, 2000, p. 4)

The problem of placement instability for foster youths has been described, in recent years, in the research literature (CWLA, 2002b; Eckenrode, Rowe, Laird, & Brathwaite, 1995). One report stated that "The first foster care placement is rarely the last. Usually, finding a permanent arrangement takes many months, if not years. Too often, it doesn't happen at all" (Youth Transition Funders Group, 2004, p. 9).

The creation of stable, permanent homes for foster youths, particularly those youths who have challenging behaviors, is not an easy task. Minimally, it requires a placement process that does not rely exclusively on a single social worker left to make decisions on his or her own with limited resources available, a short timeline, and too high a caseload. The ability to provide in-depth analysis of the child's needs and then marshal targeted, appropriate, and high quality placement options and interventions is an essential goal, one that requires funding, that supports models where children can remain with their parents, when possible, rather than be placed in out-of-home care.

Placement Process

A current model that seeks to change the traditional way CPS makes placement decisions for foster youths is the Annie E. Casey Foundation's Family to Family Initiative, which currently is being implemented in communities across twenty-two states (Family to Family, 2001). This initiative focuses on four core strategies as a way to create placement stability for foster youths and to keep them, if it is in their best interest to do so, in their home communities. These strategies include recruitment, training, and support of resource families; team decision making; building community partnerships; and self-evaluation.

The Family to Family model relies on team decision making (TDM) to determine where a child should live when considering the removal of a child from the home of an allegedly abusive or neglectful parent. A TDM meeting also is convened whenever other placement changes are contemplated including those to reunify the family, if the child has been removed. A TDM team includes the child's parent, the current caregiver, if that is not the parent, the social worker, a trained TDM facilitator from CPS, as well as others whom the parent would like to have at the meeting either because of their knowledge of the family or to provide support. Others may be included on the team by

CPS for their specific expertise, such as mental health professionals or education representatives.

Although CPS has the final say about whether the child should be removed from the home and, if so, where the child will be placed, the TDM process focuses on the strengths of the family, whether it would be safe to leave the child in the home, what supports might be needed in doing so, and, if there is a need for removal from the home, then whether there are relatives or others in the community with whom the child might live safely. The TDM team also is encouraged to consider the child's education and other needs in making a placement decision.

An important facet of the TDM process is that it does not leave the social worker to make difficult placement decisions by himself or herself. The team approach is thought to do a better job of screening children being considered for removal from home, bringing those in group or institutional care back to their neighborhoods, and involving foster families as team members in efforts to reunify families (Reed & Karpilow, 2002).

Placement Options That Keep Families Together

The Family-to-Family Initiative seeks to increase the number of foster and adoptive families within communities where there are high numbers of foster youths. This is done through the core strategy of re-cruitment, training, and support of foster and resource families. This strategy is particularly important given that the number of foster homes has decreased nationally over the last decade. This has been especially true for foster families of color and for homes that have the capacity to care for sibling groups, medically fragile infants, non-English speaking children, and children with other special needs (Reed & Karpilow, 2002). Since families are coming into the child welfare system with more severe and complex problems than ever before (Reed & Karpilow, 2002), there is a need for a wider range of living options to meet the needs of youths and families with significant challenges. Intensive support for families so that children may remain at home or be placed out-of-home, yet remain with their families, must loom larger in the repertoire of placement options available.

Building community partnerships, another Family to Family core strategy, helps to increase the network of supports and services within communities. This is important when expanding the types of residential options and services that are needed to keep families together, including high quality wraparound services, shared family care, and other supportive living alternatives.

The cases of John, Robert, and James involved youths who may have been able to remain with their birth mothers if there had been other placement options for them than those that in fact existed. Sharon might have been able to remain with her legal guardian if intensive, supportive services were available to them.

Wraparound Services

John and Robert's mothers did not know how to set appropriate limits for their difficult sons and used excessive punishment to do so, which lead to the removal of their sons from their custody. Robert's mother, for a short period of time, received in-home counseling with a therapist who set up and oversaw a behavior management system that was effective in controlling Robert's misbehavior. This was a positive step but the service was discontinued too quickly and Robert's mother reverted to her old habits of physical punishment, which were not effective and, swiftly, landed Robert in the CPS system.

John and Robert's mothers most likely could have benefited from a strong wraparound services model that provided intensive and ongoing in-home support by a counselor or therapist with expertise in positive behavior interventions. The therapists could have set up behavior intervention plans that were effective in managing the difficult behaviors of the boys, which included interventions that the mothers could have managed successfully, with intensive training, support, and oversight. Each of these mothers also could have used ongoing respite services so they could have had regular periods of time away from their sons in order to rejuvenate themselves (see Exhibit 12.2).

Sharon was living with a foster mother who had become her legal guardian. When Sharon's behavior became too erratic and difficult for her guardian to handle, she terminated the guardianship and Sharon reentered the foster care system, moving then from one failed placement to another. It clearly would have been beneficial for Sharon if her guardian had the option of receiving wraparound services to help her contend with Sharon's difficult behavior. Sharon's guardian was

EXHIBIT 12.2.
Wraparound

Wraparound is a philosophy of care that includes a definable planning process involving the child and family that results in a unique set of community services and natural supports individualized for that child and family to achieve a positive set of outcomes. (Burns & Goldman, 1999, p. 13)

not good at setting limits for her and could have benefited significantly, as would John and Robert's mothers, from intensive in home services to help her set up and effectively use an appropriate positive behavior management system.

David's long-term foster mother could have benefited from a wraparound approach as well when she no longer felt capable or willing to continue to deal with David's difficult and disturbing behavior. Instead of sending David out into the revolving door of foster care placements, he could have remained with the woman whom he considered his mother and together they could have had services that might have allowed him to remain in her home.

Wraparound is an approach to treatment that helps families with the most challenging children to function more effectively in the home, school, and community. It is an alternative to out-of-home placement. The child remains with the family and necessary supports and services are "wrapped around them" to promote success, safety, and permanence.

The wraparound process involves ongoing planning that result in individualized, comprehensive community services, and natural supports for youth with complicated, multidimensional problems and for their families. The parents and the child are integral members of the planning team to help identify the supports and services they need and evaluate their ongoing effectiveness. Wraparound has been implemented in the mental health, education, child welfare, and juvenile justice systems (Burchard, Burns, & Burchard, 2002; see Exhibit 12.3).

Policies and legislation at the federal and state levels are needed to support the wraparound philosophy and practice along with the

EXHIBIT 12.3.
Essential Elements of Wraparound Services

1. Wraparound must be based in the community
2. Services and supports must be individualized, built on strengths, and meet the needs of children and families across life domains to promote success, safety, and permanence in home, school, and community
3. The process must be culturally competent, building on the unique values, preferences, and strengths of children and families, and their communities
4. Families must be full and active partners in every level of the wrap around process
5. The wraparound approach must be a team-driven process involving the family, child, natural supports, agencies, and community services working together to develop, implement, and evaluate the individualized service plan
6. Wraparound child and family teams must have adequate, flexible approaches, and flexible funding
7. Wraparound plans must include a balance of formal services and informal community and family resources
8. In unconditional commitment to serve children and families is essential
9. The plan should be developed and implemented based on an inter agency, community-based collaborative process
10. Outcomes must be determined and measured for the system, for the program, and for the individual child and family. (Burns & Goldman, 1999, p. 14)

development of integrated service systems, funding streams, and quality assurance mechanisms (Burns & Goldman, 1999). Wraparound services for foster families require flexible interagency funding and service delivery. CPS, departments of mental health, and other state and local agencies may join together, along with community-based organizations, and blend funds to provide such services.

Studies evaluating wraparound consistently point to overall positive outcomes (Burns & Goldman, 1999). Results in two randomized studies show more positive outcomes for those involved in wraparound programs. These outcomes include fewer placement changes; greater decline in behavioral symptoms; lower overall impairment;

improvement in social, school, and community functioning; and greater likelihood of achieving permanency in the community (Burchard, Burns, & Burchard, 2002).

Shared Family Care

If wraparound services were not adequate for keeping John and Robert safely with their mothers, then another option that might have been successful—prior to placing them in out-of-home care—is shared family care. This option temporarily places an entire family, or a mother and son in the case of John and Robert, in the home of a host family that has been trained to mentor and support the biological parents as they develop skills and supports that are necessary to care for their children (Barth, 1994; Bower, 2003; Simmel & Price, 2002).

At a time when the traditional child welfare system appears to be failing in many areas and reentry rates may be as high as 30 percent (Goerge, Wulczcyn, & Harden, 1994), some within the child welfare community are attracted to the shared family care placement option (Barth, 1994; Bower, 2003; Simmel & Price, 2002). Results from small studies are promising (Bower, 2003). Children whose families complete the program are only half as likely to reenter the child welfare system as those whose families reunite after foster care. The number of participant parents (mostly mothers with jobs) doubles after they have lived with a mentor. Living conditions for these families once they are on their own are much improved. If either wraparound services or shared family care were available, neither John nor Robert would have had to experience the terrible grief, lack of self-esteem, and ultimately anger that they did at being wrenched away from their mothers' homes and care.

Residential/Group Home Placement for Child and Parent

James' mother, because of her substance abuse, needed a different placement option than John and Robert's mothers. After successfully completing a drug rehabilitation program, she quickly lost her resolve and ability to remain drug free once she was out on her own, managing the complexities of a difficult life with all the old temptations. James suffered enormously and his depression turned to rage because of his mother's failure to remain drug-free and provide him the home that he desperately needed. She could have benefited from a structured residential facility placement with strong alcohol and drug treatment available (Barth, 2002), where James and his brother could have lived with her as well.

Funding Considerations

Federal funding for CPS provides significantly more money to support foster and adoptive families than birth parents, making it more difficult to fund services to resolve crises before children are removed from their parents' home and placed in out-of-home care (Bower, 2003). Some states and local CPS agencies have sought waivers under the Child Welfare Demonstrations Projects provision authorized by Congress in 1994 (Reed & Karpilow, 2002). These waivers have allowed CPS to use Title IV-E foster care maintenance funding for innovative prevention interventions, including providing funding to implement interventions for high-risk families that do not require removing the child from the home. Clearly, more innovative placement options need to be developed and evaluated using not only safety criteria but also measures of a child's well-being.

Out-of-Home Placement Options

Foster Homes for Sibling Groups

Carlos did not have the option of remaining with his parents but needed a foster home where he and his sister Silvia could have been placed together. Carlos and Silvia were placed in different foster homes in different parts of the county, and for long periods were unable to visit each other or even talk on the telephone. After Carlos had a series of failed placements because of his behavior problems, Silvia talked her foster mother into taking Carlos into her home.

After many years of being separated and experiencing deteriorating mental health, Carlos started to thrive when he moved into the foster home where Silvia lived. For Carlos, the most sensible thing would have been to place him in the same home as his sister from the start. Then he would have had the support that he needed to survive what was for him an exceedingly difficult situation.

Therapeutic Foster Care

If any of the children could not have remained with their mothers, guardians, or long-term foster parents in the alternative placement options previously described, a better option for them, instead of placing them in the group home settings they were in, would likely have been therapeutic foster care (sometimes called treatment foster care). This option is considered the least restrictive form of out-of-home therapeutic placement for children with severe emotional disorders. Care is delivered in private homes with specially trained foster parents. Foster parents are seen as members of a treatment team, receiving specialized training and intensive support by a foster care agency, include the child and his or her family in the treatment, and receive compensation at rates higher than traditional foster care but less than the cost of residential treatment.

Research indicates that most of children in therapeutic foster care homes complete their course of treatment without a placement disruption, demonstrate improvement in social/psychological adjustment and behavior, and are discharged to less restrictive settings (Chamberlain, 2000; Curtis, Alexander, & Lunghofer, 2001; Hudson, Nutter, & Galaway, 1994; Reddy & Pfeiffer, 1997). There is evidence that therapeutic foster care is able to serve children with quite severe emotional or behavioral problems (Berrick, Courtney, & Barth, 1993; Chamberlain, 2000; Curtis et al., 2001; Hudson et al., 1994).

IMPROVING SCHOOL OUTCOMES

Children in the foster care system are among the most educationally at-risk populations of children. Foster youths are more likely than are other children to have academic and behavioral trouble in school (Altshuler, 2003). They have higher rates of absenteeism and tardiness, are more likely than other children to repeat a grade, have lower standardized test scores, and receive special education services in much higher numbers than do other children (Altshuler, 2003; Fanshel, Finch, & Grundy, 1989; Goerge et al., 1992; Parrish et al., 2001; Zima, Bussing, Freeman, Yang, Belin, & Forness, 2002).

A disproportionate number of foster children enter school with significant educational delays and they never catch up (Smithgall,

Gladen, Howard, Goerge, & Courtney, 2004). Studies find that maltreated children have more academic difficulties when compared to their nonmaltreated peers in part because they experience relatively high levels of residential mobility and school transfers (Eckenrode, et al., 1995). This school mobility leads to (1) an increase in social isolation and loss of social support associated with separations from family, friends, neighbors, schoolmates, and teachers; (2) changes in the child's affective state, which could be associated with learning difficulties; (3) discontinuities in the curriculum and teacher expectations; and (4) changes in the affective states of parents or siblings that may represent a stressor for the child (Eckenrode et al., 1995; McMillen, Auslander, Elze, White, & Thompson, 2003).

School Instability

Foster children spend a significant amount of time out of school (Parrish et al., 2001). This typically occurs when they change homes and then no longer live within the boundaries of the school they had been attending, thus requiring a change of school placement. David moved into a new foster home in a new school district and the school in that district refused to enroll him. One of the reasons for this refusal was that the new school did not have David's records from his previous school. John and Debra also ran into problems when enrolling in school. The school districts into which they moved claimed they did not have appropriate special education services for them, requiring these youngsters to be referred to county education programs. The referral process to the county programs took several months and the children were out of school for the entire time. An added problem for Debra was that she moved into her new district in the summer, when most of the district special education administrators were off and many special education programs were not operating.

AB490

In California, the legislature passed a bill, known as AB490 (2003), to address some of the problems related to schooling that foster youths face. One problem AB490 addresses is foster youths being out of school for long periods whenever they move into new home placements that are not within the boundaries of the schools they have been attending. Under this law, if a foster child or a child under the supervision of a probation department moves to a new foster or group home placement that is in a different school district from the one the child has been attending, the child may remain in the school of origin (that is, the school the child has been attending) for the remainder of the academic school year, provided it is in his or her best interest to do so. The child, and the person who holds the education rights for the child, and the school foster care liaison determine what is in the child's best interest. AB490 requires each local education agency to have a foster care liaison.

In addition, when a school change is made related to a child's move to a new foster or group home, a child is entitled to immediate enrollment in the new school. Even if the youth is unable to produce records or clothing normally required for enrollment (such as academic or medical records, immunizations, proof of residency, or school uniforms), the new school district must enroll the foster youth in the new school immediately. Had AB490 been in effect in their state when David, Debra, and John moved into their respective foster and group homes, the school districts as well as the county education agency would have been obligated under this law to immediately enroll them in school.

Inappropriate School Programs

All of the children were, at some time during their representation by Advocacy Services, in school programs that were not meeting their needs. Some of the programs were extremely inadequate. We, at Advocacy Services, spent considerable time trying to bring about changes in school programs for the children. This involved reviewing their school records, observing them in their classes, attending IEP meetings on their behalf, representing them in special education mediations, among many other activities.

Many social workers participate as much as they are able to in educational meetings of foster children on their caseloads. But few are trained well enough or have sufficient time to engage in the activities that are really necessary to ensure that foster youths are placed in appropriate school classrooms and receive necessary school services.

Education Liaison Model

The Education Liaison Model has been successful in supporting social workers in this area (Zetlin, Weinberg, & Shea, 2006b; Weinberg, Zetlin, & Kimm, 2004). The model is a comprehensive interagency program to support social workers in obtaining appropriate educational services for children in the foster care system (see Exhibit 12.4). It is a research-based model that places education liaisons in CPS offices, provides ongoing training and support to social workers in identifying educational barriers to learning and fashioning effective solutions, and provides training and technical assistance to the education liaisons so that they have sufficient expertise to resolve a wide range of complex educational problems brought to them by social workers.

Evaluation data document the effectiveness of the Education Liaison Model for both social workers and the children on their caseloads (Zetlin, 2003; Zetlin & Weinberg, 2004; Zetlin, Weinberg, & Kimm, 2005; Zetlin, Weinberg, & Kimm 2004; Zetlin, Weinberg, & Shea, 2006b; Zetlin, Weinberg, & Luderer, 2004; Zetlin, Weinberg, & Tunick, 2002). The model has been effective in (1) increasing the level of knowledge of social workers about educational procedures and programs for supporting the educational needs of foster youths; (2) increasing the social workers' level of participation in the educational process of the children on their caseloads; (3) increasing the social workers documentation of up-to-date education information included in the children's files; and (4) improving math and reading achievement test scores of children served by the education liaisons. Variants of the Education Liaison Model, where liaisons or specialists work with social workers, has been introduced and found valuable in many jurisdictions (Litchfield, Gatowski, & McKissick, 2002).

EXHIBIT 12.4.
Education Liaison Model

The Education Liaison Model is a comprehensive interagency program to support social workers in obtaining appropriate educational services for children in the foster care system. (Weinberg et al., 2004)

Lack of School Readiness

Over 30 percent of all children in the foster care system are under the age of five. Infants account for one out of every five young children who enter foster care and they remain in care twice as long as older foster children (Dicker, Gordon, & Knitzer, 2001). However, there has been relatively little attention focused on early education and intervention for these children, even though such strategies have the clear potential to reduce their risks and strengthen their families.

Infants and toddlers in foster care may show signs of attachment disorders. Preschool age foster children may be aggressive, or show signs of anxiety or depression. Over half of the young children in foster care have developmental delays (Dicker, Gordon, & Knitzer, 2001). Such delays clearly were evident in Debra and Anthony's cases.

Too many young foster children do not receive early education services that address their special needs. Most of the children described in this book did not attend preschool. Neither Anthony nor presumably Debra received any early intervention services, even though disabilities were apparent early on. Lack of enrollment in high quality early childhood education experiences is the typical pattern for many young foster children (Dicker et al., 2001). Many CPS agencies do not require caregivers to send young foster children to preschool (Zetlin et al., 2006a) and eligibility criteria for early intervention services are not well understood.

Recent studies demonstrate the importance of early childhood education for children from low-income families, of which children in foster care are highly represented (Dicker et al., 2001; Holzman, 2005; Ramey & Ramey, 2004; Rand Corporation, 1997; Rand Corporation, 2005). These studies show that preschool attendance improves children's academic achievement scores, lowers the likelihood of children repeating grades or requiring special education services, and increases the probability that children will complete high school. Studies also have shown that preschool has positive effects on lowering adolescent and adult involvement with the criminal justice systems and improving employment rates and earning average during adulthood (Rand Corporation, 2005).

Data from specially designed preschool programs for young foster children and their families have shown that disturbed and abused children can make marked improvement in development and behavior in a secure, structured therapeutic environment. Participation in these programs has enabled the children to enter the public school system for kindergarten, rather than be placed in residential facilities. Furthermore, one to five years after attending a therapeutic preschool, a high percentage of the children had improved or remained in their original type of public school classroom and had not repeated a grade (Gootman, 1996).

Head Start and Early Head Start

Head Start is a free, federally funded program for preschool children—three to five years old from low-income families. Head Start programs are operated by local nonprofit organizations in almost every county in the country. The program provides educational, family development, social and health (including nutrition and mental health) services, and transportation. Early Head Start, for infants and children of ages birth to three, provides high-quality child and family development services.

Foster children are eligible to attend Head Start programs and the programs must be comprised of at least 10 percent of children with disabilities. Data indicate that only 6 percent of foster children under six attend Head Start (Vandivere, Chalk, & Moore, 2003). This may be because there are not enough spaces for all the children who want to attend and foster children are not typically given the priority status to which they may be entitled (Zetlin et al., 2006a). Furthermore, many of the programs are only half day, making it difficult for caregivers who work outside the home to have the children in their care attend.

There are, however, Head Start and Early Head Start programs that specifically focus on the needs of foster children, such as West Boone Early Head Start (Dicker et al., 2001). The goal of the program is to enhance the child's development and promote reunification for the child with the biological parents. An individualized plan is developed for each family, with most families spending five days each week in the program where they learn about child development, health, nutrition, and safety, and participate in the attachment and bonding program. The program includes mental health consultations for the parent and child, clinical supervision, and home visits. Two of the children described in this book—specifically, John and Robert—along with their mothers, very likely would have benefited significantly from this type of Early Head Start program.

Early Intervention Services

Young children, between the ages of birth and three, with diagnosed conditions resulting in developmental delays (e.g., cerebral palsy, Down syndrome), documented delays (e.g., in cognitive development, social/emotional development, communication), or, in some states, conditions that are at high risk for substantial developmental delay (e.g., prenatal substance abuse; thirty-two-week gestation) are entitled to receive publicly funded early intervention services under the IDEA Act (2004). Services may include special instruction for the children (e.g., infant stimulation or preschool programs), family training, psychological counseling, respite services for caregivers, and transportation designed to meet the developmental needs of the child or family. Those entitled to receive services include the child, the parents, including biological and adoptive parents, a relative with whom the child lives, a legal guardian, and, in some states, a foster parent and other caregivers, and others in order to enhance the development of the child. The IDEA (2004) specifically requires that all children under age three who have substantiated cases of abuse or neglect are to be referred for early intervention services.

Other Preschool Programs

Other early education services specifically designed for foster children include Kempe early education project serving abused families (KEEPSAFE), a therapeutic preschool and home visitation program for three- to six-year-old children and their families (Gootman, 1996; Gray, 2000). Through the use of a therapeutic classroom, a psychologically safe environment is created where each child is exposed to a daily and weekly routine, consistent limits and rules, choice making, repetition of activities, consistent staff, and a teacher/ case manager who is also responsible for home visits. The curriculum focuses on the knowledge and preacademic skills required for entry into public school. Each child sees an individual psychotherapist for

weekly or twice weekly sessions and participates in daily group therapy sessions focused on issues such as safety and hygiene. The parent
component has two goals: (1) to give caretakers emotional support
from staff members and referrals to other psychological services; and
(2) to improve the quality of the interaction between the child and caregiver. This type of early education program might have provided John
and his mother a good foundation for further development.

Lack of Intensive Academic Skill Development

Many foster youth leave the foster care system without basic literacy skills, leaving them ill prepared for adult life (Youth Transition
Funders Group, 2004). Silvia at age fifteen and Carlos at age nine
could not read. David also struggled with reading. Such children
need intense, effective programs to develop their reading skills.

Researchers have identified why most special education placements
are not more effective in bringing the reading skills of students the ages
of Carlos, Silvia, and David into the average range within a reasonable
period of time (Vaughn, Moody, & Shuman, 1998). The interventions
do not have sufficient intensity because teachers are responsible for
too many students and are not able to offer individualized instruction.
Furthermore, there is little direct instruction or guided practice in
such critical areas as phonemic awareness, phonemic decoding, and
comprehension strategies.

Studies of intensive interventions with older children with reading
disabilities demonstrate that it is possible to accelerate their reading
growth to a much greater extent than is typically achieved in special
education classrooms (Torgesen, 2005). The principles of instruction
that have generally been found to be successful for children with reading disabilities include: (1) ample opportunities for guided practice of
new skills, (2) very intensive instruction, (3) systematic cueing of appropriate strategies in reading words or text, and (4) explicit instruction
in phonemic decoding strategies (Swanson, 1999). Torgesen recom-
mends that for students who are about two years below grade level
by the fourth or fifth grade, they should have three-hour blocks of
daily reading instruction. In addition to implementing more effective
strategies for older children, it is also essential to focus more of our
instructional resources on preventing the emergence of reading dis-

abilities in children who are just beginning to learn to read. Hopefully, the language in the IDEA (2004) and its implementing regulations regarding early identification and the provision of effective, research-based interventions within general education will provide effective remediation of early reading problems for young foster children.

Tutoring sometimes is offered to foster youths who are not achieving adequately in school. It is important to distinguish intensive skill building in subject matter areas from tutoring. Tutoring to help students on homework or to study for tests will not necessarily provide the intensive academic skill building that a great many foster youth need in reading, mathematics, or writing. However, some tutoring models have been shown to be effective.

Treehouse Tutoring Program

The Treehouse Tutoring Program was established in Seattle, Washington in a number of elementary schools that serve high numbers of foster children in out-of-home placement. The tutors are housed in the elementary schools and meet on a daily basis with the students who have been referred to them by their social workers. The tutors begin by building trust and becoming a dependable adult in the child's life. They also meet regularly with teachers to set academic and behavioral goals for the students and to alert teachers to the foster care status and unique needs of the children, such as their high risk for memory problems, attention difficulties, sleep and mood disorders, emotional problems and chronic health problems such as asthma and malnutrition. Evaluation results from this program have been positive. Of the sixty-five children served by Treehouse tutors over one school year, only two students did not advance to the next grade level. More than half improved their math, reading, and spelling skills by one or more grade levels. More than two thirds met all or most of their individual behavioral goals and most of them met all or most of their reading and math goals (Jacobson, 1998; Teichroeb, 1999).

IMPROVING MENTAL HEALTH OUTCOMES

A substantial proportion of children in the foster care system exhibit emotional and behavioral disorders and have much higher rates of these disorders than do children from their same socioeconomic background (Committee on Early Childhood, Adoption, and Dependent Care, American Academy of Pediatrics, 2002). Some studies indicate that between 40 and 60 percent of youths in foster care have at least one psychiatric disorder, and approximately 33 percent have three or more diagnosed psychiatric conditions (dos Reis, Zito, Safer, & Soeken, 2001). A review of case records of older foster youths who had been discharged from out-of-home placement revealed that 67 percent of these youths met the criteria for a psychiatric disorder and 44 percent had been in a psychiatric hospital (McCann, James, Wilson, & Dunn, 1996).

All of the children described in this book had emotional or behavioral disorders. Some at the mild to moderate level, such as Silvia, Carlos, and Anthony, and others, like Sharon, John, James, Robert, Debra, Patty, and David at the moderate to severe level. The problem for these children was that it was almost impossible for them to receive the therapeutic support they needed on an ongoing basis. It was hard for some, such as Silvia and Carlos, to access mental health services at all. For others, their services were inconsistent as they moved from placement to placement. John and Robert did not have mental health services in place when, for a short period of time, they were placed back in the homes of their mothers, leading to the quick demise of a trial home-of-parent placement. None of the children, who were placed at the county emergency shelter, were able to access mental health services through the special education process, which was the only real entitlement to mental health services that existed.

Other problems the children faced included lack of consistent mental health treatment. Some of them received frequent psychological evaluations from different evaluators, often with quite disparate results. Some of the evaluations were excellent; others were extremely cursory with little attention paid to the background and experiences of the children. The mental health clinicians the children saw for psychological therapy changed constantly. Frequently, these clinicians were novices in the field who had little background or experience to contend with the severe, entrenched, mental health problems these children had.

Inconsistent and changing psychiatric treatment sometimes led to a haphazard way of determining what psychotropic medication was appropriate to treat the particular psychiatric disorders the children had. And as they moved from placement to placement, with different psychiatrists diagnosing their disorders and prescribing medication with each placement change, the medications were constantly being changed. Psychiatrists frequently were given little or no information about medications previously tried and the side effects that had occurred.

High Quality Assessments and Treatment

Children entering foster care should receive high quality, periodic assessments of their emotional and behavioral status (Clausen et al., 1998). Evaluators with training and expertise with this population of children should perform the assessments. The assessors should be part of mental health treatment teams that oversee or provide ongoing psychological or psychiatric care to the children. The treatment teams must be knowledgeable about the psychological problems of youths in foster care. They also should oversee the psychological therapy and psychiatric treatment when the youths are in settings where other mental health practitioners provide their therapeutic treatment. This team should make appropriate referrals to various treatment modalities, when appropriate, including early intervention services for children between birth and three. Other needed services are those specifically designed to target deficits in social competency and adaptive behavior, such as group psychotherapy, recreational interventions, and social skills building (Clausen et. al., 1998).

Given the high prevalence of mental health problems in foster youth, research suggests that preventive approaches designed to promote social skills, self-regulation, and coping bring about positive outcomes (Harden, 2004). Interventions that help foster parents better support the emotional needs of youth in their care also have shown success (Fisher, Gunner, Chamberlain, & Reid, 2000).

CREATING STABLE TRANSITION TO ADULTHOOD

Many youths leave foster care without the support systems and skills to guide them into productive adulthood (Weinberg, Zetlin, &

Shea, 2001). Studies have found that between one third and two thirds of current or former foster youth dropout before completing high school, or by age nineteen, have received neither a high school diploma nor a GED compared to 10 percent of their same-age peers (Blome, 1997; Courtney & Dworsky, 2005; Joiner, 2001). A study of former foster youth found that 28 percent had been arrested and almost 20 percent had been incarcerated (Courtney & Dworsky, 2005). Approximately, one in seven young women who age out of foster care report being raped (Courtney, Piliavin, & Grogan-Kaylor, 1995). In another study, 33 percent of current and former female foster youth age seventeen and eighteen report having been pregnant (Courtney, Terao, & Bost, 2004). Less than a fifth of former foster youth report receiving any job training or help in signing up for medical benefits before leaving the foster care system. Another study found that for nineteen-year-olds, who were no longer in care, almost 14 percent had been homeless and over 50 percent suffered one or more indicators of economic hardship (e.g., not having enough to eat, being evicted, phone service turned off, etc.; Courtney & Dworsky, 2005).

Independent Living/Independent Living Skills Program

In 1986, with the passage of the Independent Living Program Act (ILP), federal funding became available to help states prepare foster youth for independent living. This law allowed states to use these funds for Title IVE eligible foster youth[1] of age sixteen and older for services to promote self-sufficiency and to transition the youth out of the foster care system. In 1988, the ILP-eligible population was expanded to all sixteen- and eighteen-year-old foster youth regardless of their Title IVE status and to former foster youth who had exited foster care within the past six months. Starting in 1990, states had the option of providing ILP services to youth until age twenty-one. However, only a small number of foster youth eligible for ILP services received them (U.S. DHHS, 1999). More than a decade after the implementation of Title IVE Independent Living Programs, what little evidence exists indicates that foster youth largely are unprepared for independent living upon leaving the foster care system as young adults. As a result, in 1999, Congress passed the Foster Care Independence Act, doubling yearly funding to states for independent living skills programs (ILSP), allowing states to use some funding for transitional living programs for emancipated youth, and to extend Medicaid coverage to age twenty-one so that youth leaving foster care would continue to have medical coverage. The services available to youth include educational support, employment services or training, budget and financial management services, health education services, help finding and maintaining housing, and services to promote youth development.

None of the children age fourteen or older described in this book was provided ILP or ILSP services. CPS reserved their limited number of ILP and ILSP spaces for youth without disabilities or behavior problems. Consequently, Advocacy Services attorneys employed other strategies to help the youth prepare for their lives after foster care.

Individual Transition Plan

Pam, Advocacy Services' staff attorney, spent considerable time trying to weave together a transition program for Robert, who at the time was living at the county emergency shelter. Since he was nearing the time he would "age out" of foster care, Pam wanted him to develop vocational and other independent living skills and have services in place so that when he left the system, he would have a means of support, a place to live, vocational opportunities, and other needed support services. Pam used the Individual Transition Plan (ITP), a required component of the IEP for students receiving special education services age sixteen and older, to bring needed agencies together to plan for Robert's future. Nancy, Advocacy Services' senior attorney, also used the ITP as a mechanism to bring appropriate agencies together for Patty when she was ready to transition from her residential program to a living situation when she no longer would be in foster care (see Exhibit 12.5).

For foster youth, it is important that there be coordination between the ILSP services provided by CPS and the transition services provided by the school district. CPS should be invited to participate in a foster youth's ITP meeting so that services can be properly coordinated.

EXHIBIT 12.5.
Individual Transition Plan

Under the IDEA, transition services are defined as a coordinated set of activities for a student with a disability that:

1. promote movement from school to post school activities, including post-secondary education, vocational training, employment, and independent living
2. are based on the students need's taking into account the student's preferences and interests and
3. include instruction, related services, community experiences, the development of employment and other post-school adult living objectives, and when appropriate, acquisition of daily living skills and functional vocational evaluation. (IDEA, 2004)

Recent Initiatives

Youth Transition Funders Groups

In recent years, increased attention has focused on the needs of transition-age foster youth and the grim statistics of those leaving the foster care system as adults. Leaders from private foundations interested in improving the lives of vulnerable youth contend that for foster youth to become successful adults requires intensive coordinated efforts of many organizations and individuals to provide the support and encouragement these young people need to become engaged, responsible, and productive adults (Youth Transition Funders Group, 2004). They argue: "It requires that they have a community-wide network of connections and support that can provide pathways to life-long economic well-being and financial success." (p. 15). In order to put together this network, the foundation leaders have issued reports and invested in a comprehensive initiative to support the transition of foster youth to adult life. The initiative includes components to (1) advocate and support educational attainment; (2) facilitate access to workforce development opportunities; (3) provide financial literacy education, (4) encourage savings and asset development; and (5) create entrepreneurship opportunities (Youth Transition Funders Group, 2004). Demonstration communities for the initiative must include the following program elements: a debit card account, a matched savings account, financial literacy education, an educational advocate, youth leadership opportunities, and "door opener" opportunities.

Foster Youth Transition Project

The Foster Youth Transition Project (FYTP)[2] provides financial support and technical assistance to a small cohort of California Family to Family Initiative counties to develop a comprehensive continuum of services to support foster youth, ages fourteen to twenty-four, who are transitioning to adulthood. Counties receive $300,000 over three years to implement plans developed through county self-assessments. The counties consider the following questions during the FYTP planning process:

- How are we partnering with local workforce investment boards, businesses, community colleges, institutions of higher education, and community partners to create sector-specific training and career pathways that link older foster youth with jobs in growing industries?
- What partnerships have we formed with public and private housing providers to expand supportive housing options for foster youth?
- How are we working with the local school district to improve educational outcomes for foster youth?
- How are we partnering with public agency and community-based organizations to build personal and social assets for foster youth that support positive, physical, psychological, emotional, and social development?
- How are we developing lifelong relationships between foster youth and caring, committed, loving adults?
- How do our core training programs empower families, youth, foster parents, group homes, foster family agencies, kinship families, guardians, and agency staff to meet the needs of emancipating foster youth?
- How is the Independent Living Skills Program (ILSP) integrated within all levels of our agency? Are ILSP services accessible to foster youth?

Many of the children described in this book could have benefited from the programs developed by the communities funded to implement these initiatives. However, it is essential that these programs have the capability to serve the type of children described in this book and to link these services to the children's ITP.

Children's Village Work Appreciation for Youth (WAY)

The Children's Village WAY Program, an Independent Living Program, provides a paid-professional mentor for older foster youth who transition out of the foster care system and out of the program's residential treatment center (RTC) (Baker, Olson, & Mincer, 2000). Children's Village studied the outcomes for those who left the RTC program between 1989 and 1995, all of whom were between the ages of twenty-one and thirty at the time of the study. They were nearly all from impoverished communities and had been special education students when they came to Children's Village. Sixty-six percent were African American and 27 percent were Hispanic. The studies showed that 80 percent of the RTC youth who had been in the WAY Program had graduated high school, earned a GED, or were still in school. These results are dramatically better than graduation statistics on comparable groups. Eighty percent of WAY alumni who had been a part of the study were employed. Only 8 percent had been arrested for violent crimes since age twenty-one.

In addition to providing a paid mentor, the WAY Program also offers work experience, individual counseling, work ethics instruction, tutoring, financial incentives for saving, and a five-year commitment to youth leaving foster care. Longitudinal data indicate that none of the 300 youths who have been through the program were on welfare and over half of them went on to postsecondary education (Baker et al., 2000).

AB408

Debra, Patty, and David were without any familial support. This situation, unfortunately, is the norm for many foster youths. Upon exiting the foster care system, foster youths frequently lack relationships with caring adults who can help them navigate the difficult transition into adult life. Legislation, known as AB408, enacted into law in 2003 in California, attempts to address this deficiency by requiring CPS social workers to ask every child over the age of ten, who has been in foster care for at least six months and has been placed in a group home, to identify individuals "who are important to the child," and to provide this information in court reports and case plans (*AB 408*, §366.1(g)). For children under age ten, social workers must make the same inquiry "as appropriate." In addition to requiring social workers to ask children about the adults important to them, AB408 also requires that social workers help youth maintain these relationships and report to the court on the actions they have taken to do so. AB408 also allows the state's Independent Living Program to allocate resources to strengthen the relationships. AB408 would have aided David in maintaining his relationship with the foster mother he thought of as his mother and Sharon with the woman who had been her legal guardian.

FINAL THOUGHTS

This final chapter has focused on crucial areas where change is needed to better provide for one of our most vulnerable populations of children. It has not meant to be exhaustive in terms of covering every possible change that has been suggested in the literature. Rather, the cases of the children that comprise the heart of this book have dictated the recommendations for change, based on the identified cracks in the multiagency system of care. Strong advocacy is always needed for these children. However, as the book reveals, advocacy, while essential, is not always able to deliver the foundation these youth need to grow into educated, healthy, and productive adults.

SUMMARY

The purpose of this chapter was to look closely at the cracks revealed by the case studies of the children described in this book in the multiagency system of care, responsible for proving them stable living environments, appropriate schooling, and supportive mental health and other services. The chapter not only reveals the cracks but also describes interventions and systemic policy changes that could help repair many of them.

Notes

Preface

1. All of the children have been given fictitious names and facts about them have been altered to maintain their confidentiality.

2. This is not the real name of the private, nonprofit law firm that represented the children.

Chapter 1

1. Pellman (1996) defines judicial officers as referees, commissioners, and judges. I use the term "judge" in the remainder of the book for purposes of clarity and consistency.

Chapter 2

1. For children ages three to nine, a state may elect to simply identify the student as a "child with a disability" in order to qualify for special education services. 20 U.S.C. §1402(1)(B).

Chapter 12

1. Youth who are Title IVE eligible are those placed in the foster care system by a court order and who meet eligibility requirements of the Aid to Families with Dependent Children (AFDC) program.

2. The Foster Youth Transition Project is supported by the Annie E. Casey Foundation Family to Family Initiative, the Stuart Foundation, and the Walter S. Johnson Foundation.

The Systematic Mistreatment of Children in the Foster Care System
© 2007 by The Haworth Press, Taylor & Francis Group. All rights reserved.
doi:10.1300/5136_13

311

References

AB 408 (2003). Cal. Welf. & Inst. Code §366.1(g); §10609.4(b)(1)(G).

AB 490 (2003). An act to amend Sections 48645.5, 48850, 48859, 49061, 49069.5, 49076, and 56055 of, and to add Sections 48853 and 48853.5 to, the Calif. Educ. Code, and to amend Sections 361, 366.27, 726, 727.2, 4570, 16000, and 16501.1 of the Calif. Welf. & Instit. Code, relating to minors.

Admissions & Judicial Commitment, Mentally Retarded Persons. Calif. Welf. & Inst. Code Ann. §6500 (Deerings, 2003).

Adoption and Foster Care Analysis and Reporting System. (2006a). *The AFCARS report: Preliminary FY 2005 estimates as of September 2006.* Retrieved March 29, 2007, from http://www.acf.hhs.gov/programs/cb/stats_research/afcars/tar/report13.htm

Adoption and Foster Care Analysis and Reporting System. (2006b). *Trends in foster care and adoption—FY 2000-FY2005.* Retrieved March 29, 2007, from http://www.acf.hhs.gov/programs/cb/stats_research/afcars/trends.htm

Adoption and Safe Families Act of 1997, Public Law 105-89, 42 U.S.C. §§620-679.

Adoption Assistance and Child Welfare Act of 1980. PL 96-272. Amended titles IV E and IV-B of the Social Security Act, 94 Stat. 500.

Aldridge, M. & Cautley, P. (1976). Placing siblings in the same foster home. *Child Welfare, LV*(2), 85-93.

Altshuler, S. J. (2003). From barriers to successful collaborations: Public schools and child welfare working together. *Social Work, 48*(1), 52-63.

Assistance to States for the Education of Children with Disabilities. (1997). 34 C.F.R. §300.342(b)(2) including Note; 300.346.

Assistance to States for the Education of Children with Disabilities, 70 Fed. Reg. 35782 (June 21, 2005) (to be codified at 34 C.F.R. pt 300.8; 300.151).

Badeau, S. & Gesiriech, S. (2003). *A child's journey through the child welfare system.* Washington, DC: The Pew Commission on Children in Foster Care. Retrieved on March 22, 2007 at http://pewfostercare.org/docs/index.php?DocID=24

Baker, A. J. L., Olson, D., & Mincer, C. (2000). *The WAY to Work: An independent living/aftercare program for high risk youth.* Washington, DC: Child Welfare League of America.

Barth, R. P. (1994). Shared family care: Child protection and family preservation. *Social Work, 39*(5), 515-524.

Bauer, A. (1993). Children and youth in foster care. *Intervention in School and Clinic, 28,* 134-142.

The Systematic Mistreatment of Children in the Foster Care System
© 2007 by The Haworth Press, Taylor & Francis Group. All rights reserved.
doi:10.1300/5136_14

Berrick, J., Courtney, M., & Barth, R. (1993). Specialized foster care and group home care: Similarities and differences in the characteristics of children in care. *Children & Youth Services Review, 15*, 453-473.

Besharov, D. J. (1983). Protecting abused and neglected children: Can law help social work? *Child Abuse & Neglect, 7*, 421-434.

Besharov, D. J. (1985). Right versus rights: The dilemma of child protection. *Public Welfare*, 19-27.

Blome, W. (1997). What happens to foster kids: Educational experiences of a random sample of foster care youth and a matched group of non-foster care youth. *Child and Adolescent Social Work, 14*, 41-53.

Board of Education v. Holland, 4 F. 3d 1398 (9th Cir. 1994).

Bower, A. (Feb. 17, 2003). Troubled parents are getting a second chance: Foster care for them, along with their kids. *Time Magazine*, 23-26.

Burchard, J. D., Bruns, E. L., & Burchard, S. N. (2002). The wraparound approach. In B. J. Burns & K. Hoagwood (Eds.), *Community-based treatment for youth*: *Evidence-based interventions for severe emotional and behavioral disorders* (pp. 69-90). New York: Oxford University Press.

Burns, B. J. & Goldman, S. K. (Eds.) (1999). Promising practices in wraparound for children with serious emotional disturbance and their families. *Systems of Care: Promising Practices in Children's Mental Health, 1998 Series, Volume IV.* Washington, DC: Center for Effective Collaboration and Practice, American Institutes for Research. Retrieved on March 22, 2007, from http://cecp.air.org/promisingpractices/1998monographs/vol4.pdf

Carroll, C. A. & Haase, C. C. (1988). The function of protective services in child abuse and neglect. In R. E. Helfer & R. S. Kempe (Eds.), *The battered child* (4th ed., pp. 137-151). Chicago: University of Chicago.

Casey Family Programs. (2003). *Siblings in out-of-home care: An overview.* National Center for Resource Family Support. Retrieved March 22, 2007, from http://www.hunter.cuny.edu/socwork/nrcfcpp/downloads/sibling_overview.pdf

Chamberlain, P. (2000). What works in treatment foster care. In M. Kluger, G. Alexander, & P. Curtis (Eds.), *What Works in Child Welfare* (pp. 157-162). Washington, DC: Child Welfare League of America. Child Abuse Prevention and Treatment Act (1974). Amended and reauthorized in 2003. 42 U.S.C.A. §5103.

Child Abuse Prevention and Treatment Act of 1974 (CAPTA), Public Law 93-247, as amended by *Keeping Children and Families Safe Act of 2003,* Public Law 108-36, 42 U.S.C. §51006a.

Child Welfare Information Gateway. (2005a). *Definitions of child abuse and neglect.* State Statutes Series. Retrieved on March 29, 2007 at http://www.childwelfare. gov/systemwide/laws_policies/statutes/define.cfm

Child Welfare Information Gateway. (2005b). *Definitions of child abuse and neglect:* Summary of state laws. State Statutes Series. Retrieved on March 29, 2007 at http://www.childwelfare.gov/systemwide/laws_policies/statutes/defineall.pdf

Child Welfare Information Gateway. (2005c). *Mandatory reporters of child abuse and neglect: Summary of State Laws.* State Statutes Series. Retrieved on March 29, 2007 from http://www.childwelfare.gov/systemwide/laws_policies/statutes/mandaall.pdf

Child Welfare League of America. (2002a). Child welfare workforce. *Research Roundup*. Washington, DC: Author.

Child Welfare League of America. (2002b). Improving educational outcomes for youth in care: A national collaboration. *Background Paper*. Washington, DC: Author.

Child Welfare League of America. (2004). Testimony submitted to the Subcommittee on Human Resources of the Committee on Ways and Means U.S. House of Representatives for the hearing on state efforts to comply with federal child welfare reviews. Retrieved on June 10, 2004, from http:/www.cwla.org/advocacy/CFSR040513.htm

Chipunga, S. S. & Bent-Goodley, T. B. (2004). Meeting the challenges of contemporary foster care. *The Future of Children, 14*(1), 75-93.

Choice, P., D'Andrade, A., Gunther, K., Downes, D., Schaldach, J., Csiszar, C., & Austin, M.J. (2001). *Education for foster children: Removing barriers to academic success.* Berkeley: University of California, Berkeley, School of Social Welfare, Center for Social Services Research.

Clausen, J. M., Landsverk, J., Ganger, W., Chadwick, D., & Litrownik, A. (1998). Mental health problems of children in foster care. *Journal of Child and Family Studies, 7*(3), 283-296.

Committee on Early Childhood, Adoption, and Dependent Care, American Academy of Pediatrics. (March 2002). *Pediatrics, 109*(3), 536-541. Retrieved from: http://aapolicy.aapublications.org/cgi/content/full/pediatrics:109/3/536

Cook, R. J. (1994). Are we helping foster care youth prepare for their future? *Children & Youth Services Review, 16,* 213-229.

Courtney, M. E. & Dworsky, A. (2005). *Midwest evaluation of the adult functioning of former foster youth: Outcomes at age 19.* Chicago, IL: Chapin Hall Center for Children.

Courtney, M., Dworsky, A., Terao, S., Ruth, G., & Keller, T. (2005). *Midwest evaluation of the adult functioning of former foster youth.* Chicago, IL: Chapin Hall Center for Children, University of Chicago.

Courtney, M., Piliavin, I., & Grogan-Kaylor, A. (1995). *The Wisconsin study of youth aging out of out-of-home care: A portrait of children about to leave care. Report to the Wisconsin Department of Health and Social Services.* Madison, WI: School of Social Work, University of Wisconsin-Madison.

Courtney, M. E., Roderick, M., Smithgall, C., Gladden, R. M., & Nagoka, J. (2004). *The educational status of foster children.* Chicago: University of Chicago, Chapin Hall Center for Children, Issue Brief #102.

Courtney, M. E., Terao, S., & Bost, N. (2004). *Midwest evaluation of the adult functioning of former foster youth: Conditions of youth preparing to leave state care.* Chicago: Chapin Hall Center for Children at the University of Chicago.

Curtis, P., Alexander, G., & Lunghofer, L. (2001). A literature review comparing the outcomes of residential group care and therapeutic foster care. *Child and Adolescent Social Work Journal, 18*(5), 377-392.

Daniel R. R. v. El Paso Independent School District 874 F. 2d 1036 (5th Cir. 1989).

Dependent Children-Judgment and Orders, Calif. Welf. & Inst. Code §362(a) (Deerings Ann. 2006).

Developmental Disability Act of 1984 (P.L.98-527), amended and reauthorized in 1987 and 1999, P.L. 106-402, §42 USCS §6001; 6001(7).

Dicker, S., Gordon, E., & Knitzer, J. (2001). *Improving the Odd for the Healthy Development of Young Children in Foster Care.* New York: National Center for Children in Poverty.

dos Reis, S., Zito, J. M., Safer, D. J., & Soeken, K. L. (2001). *American Journal of Public Health, 91*(7), 1094-1099.

Eckenrode, J., Laird, M., & Doris, J. (1993). School performance and disciplinary problems among abused and neglected children. *Developmental Psychology, 29,* 53-62.

Eckenrode, J., Rowe, E., Laird, M., & Brathwaite, J. (1995). Mobility as a mediator of the effects of child maltreatment on academic performance. *Child Development, 66,* 1130-1142.

Faller, K. C. (1985). Unanticipated problems in the United States Child Protection System. *Child Abuse & Neglect, 9,* 63-69.

Family to Family. (2001). *Lessons learned.* Philadelphia, PA: Center for Applied Research. Retrieved March 11, 2006, from www.aecf.org/initiatives/familytofamily/tools/lessons.htm

Fanshel, D., Finch, S., & Grundy, J. (1989). Foster children in life-course perspective: The Casey family program experience. *Child Welfare, 68,* 467-478.

Fisher, P., Gunnar, M., Chamberlain, P., & Reid, J. (2000). Preventive intervention for maltreated preschool children: Impact on children's behavior, neuroendocrine activity, and foster parent functioning. *Journal of the American Academy of Child and Adolescent Psychiatry, 39,* 1356-1364.

Giangreco, M., Edelman, S., Luiselli, T., & MacFarland, S. (1997). Helping or hovering? Effects of instructional assistant proximity on students with disabilities. *Exceptional Children, 64,* 7-18.

Goerge, R. M., Voorhis, J. V., Grant, S., Casey, K., & Robinson, M. (1992). Special-education experiences of foster children: An empirical study. *Child Welfare, 71,* 419-437.

Goerge, R., Wulczcyn, F., & Harden, A. (1994). *An update from the multi-state foster care data archive: Foster care dynamics 1983-1993.* The Chapin Hall Center at the University of Chicago.

Gootman, M. E. (1996). Child abuse and its implications for early childhood educators. *Preventing School Failure, 40,* 149-154.

Gray, J. (2000). Academic progress of children who attended a preschool for abused children: A follow-up of the Keepsafe project. *Child Abuse & Neglect, 24*(1), 25-32.

Greer v. Rome City School District 950 F. 2d 688 (11th Cir. 1991).

Griswold v. Connecticut, 381 U.S. 4479 (1965).

Gunderson, D. & Osborne, S. (Winter 2001). Addressing the crisis in child welfare social worker turnover. *North Carolina Journal for Families and Children,* 2-6.

Harden, B. J. (Winter 2004). Safety and stability for foster children. A developmental perspective. *Children, Families, and Foster Care, 14*(1), 31-47.

Hingsburger, D. & Tough, S. (2002). Healthy sexuality: Attitudes, systems, and policies. *Research & Practice for Persons with Severe Disabilities, 27*(1), 8-17.

Hochstadt, N. J., Jaudes, P. K., Zimo, D. A., & Schachter, J. (1987). The medical and psychosocial needs of children entering foster care. *Child Abuse and Neglect, 11,* 53-62.

Holzman, M. (January 19, 2005). Preschools effects at 40. *Education Week,* p. 33.

House Report No. 101-544, 10 (1990).

Howing, P. T. & Wodarski, J. S. (1992). Legal requisites for social workers in child abuse and neglect situations. *Social Work, 37*(4), 330-336.

Hudson, J., Nutter, R. W., & Galaway, B. (1994). Treatment foster care programs: A review of evaluation research and suggested directions. *Social Work Research, 18*(4), 198-210.

Hughes Bill (1990) (AB 2586). Calif. Educ. Code Ann. §§56520-56524 (Deerings, 2006, 2006); 5CCR §3052.

Individuals with Disabilities Education Act (formerly the *Education for All Handicapped Children Act of 1975*), as amended by the *Individuals with Disabilities Education Act of 1997*, P.L. 105-17 (June 4, 1997) and the *Individuals with Disabilities Education Improvement Act of 2004,* P.L. 108-446 (Dec. 2004), 20 U.S.C. §1400 et seq.

Interagency Responsibilities for Related Services. (2004). Calif. Gov't Code §7570 et seq.

Jacobson, L. (1998). One on one. *Education Week, 18*(1), 42-47.

Janko, S. (1994). *Vulnerable children, vulnerable families.* New York: Teachers College, Columbia University.

Jellinek, M. S., Murphy, J. M., Poitrast, F., Gwinn, D., Bishop, S.J., & Goshko, M. (1992). Serious child mistreatment in Massachusetts: The course of 206 children through the courts. *Child Abuse & Neglect, 16,* 179-185.

Joiner, L. L. (2001). Reaching out to children in care. *American School Board Journal,* 30-37.

Jones, F. (2007). *Tools for teaching: Discipline, instruction, motivation* (2nd ed.), Santa Cruz, CA: Fredric H. Jones & Associates.

Juvenile Court Proceedings: Joinder of parties. Calif. Welf. & Inst. Code Ann. §362(a) (Deerings, 2006).

Kavale, K. A. & Forness, S. A. (2000). History, rhetoric, and reality: Analysis of the inclusion debate. *Remedial & Special Education, 21*(5), 279-296.

Kelly, K. (October 2000). The educational crisis of children in the juvenile court system. *Update, 1*(3), 1, 4-6.

Knitzer, J. (1982). *Unclaimed children.* Washington, D. C.: Children's Defense Fund.

Kurtz, P. D., Gaudin, J. M. Jr., Wodarski, J. S., & Howing, P. T. (1993). Maltreatment and the school-aged child: School performance consequences. *Child Abuse and Neglect, 17,* 581-589.

Lanterman Developmental Disabilities Services Act of 1969. Calif. Welf. & Inst. Code §4500 et seq.

Lanterman-Petris-Short Act of 1968. Calif. Welf. & Inst. Code §5150 et seq.

Lawrence, C. & Lankford, V. (1997 December). Sibling loss: The hidden tragedy of the child welfare system. *Adoptive Families.* Retrieved March 26, 2006, from http://www.nysccc.org/Siblings/hiddentragedy.htm

Leiter, J. & Johnson, M. C. (1994). Child maltreatment and school performance. *American Journal of Education, 102,* 154-189.

Leiter, J. & Johnsen, M. C. (1997). Child maltreatment and school performance declines: An event-history analysis. *American Education Research Journal, 34,* 563-589.

Lindsey, D. (2004). *The welfare of children.* NY: Oxford University Press.

Litchfield, M., Gatowksi, S. I., & McKissick, M. (2002). *Improving educational outcomes for youth in foster care: Perspectives from judges and program specialists.* Reno: National Council of Juvenile and Family Court Judges.

Marks, S. U., Schrader, C., & Levine, M. (1999). Paraeducator experiences in inclusive settings: Helping, hovering, or holding their own? *Exceptional Children, 65,* 315-328.

Mason, M. A. & Gambull, E. (1994). Limiting abuse reporting laws. In M. A. Mason & E. Gambull (Eds.), *Debating children's lives.* (p. 285). Thousand Oaks: Sage.

McCann, J. C., James, A., Wilson, S., & Dunn, G. (1996). Prevalence of psychiatric disorders in young people in the care system. *British Medical Journal, 313,* 1529-1530.

McCarthy, J., Marshall, A., Collins, J., Arganza, G., Deserly, K., & Milon, J. (2003). *A family's guide to the child welfare system.* Sponsored by the National Technical Assistance Center for Children's Mental Health at Georgetown University Center for Child and Human Development, Technical Assistance Partnership for Child and Family Mental Health at American Institutes for Research, Federation of Families for Children's Mental Health, Child Welfare League of America, and the National Indian Child Welfare Association. Retrieved March 26, 2006, from http://gucchd.georgetown.edu/files/product

McIntyre, A. & Keesler, T. Y. (1986). Psychological disorders among foster children. *Journal of Clinical Psychology, 15,* 297-303.

McKinney-Vento Homeless Assistance Act (2001). 42 USC §11431 et seq.

McMillen, C., Auslander, W., Elze, D., White, T., & Thompson, R. (2003). Educational experiences and aspirations of older youth in foster care. *Child Welfare, 82*(4), 475-495.

McMillen, J. C. & Tucker, J. (1999). The status of older adolescents at exit from out-of-home care. *Child Welfare, 78,* 339-360.

Meddin, B. J. & Hansen, I. (1985). The services provided during a child abuse and/or neglect case investigation and the barriers that exist to service provision. *Child Abuse & Neglect, 9,* 175-182.

Meyer v. Nebraska, 262 U.S. 390 (1963).

Miller v. Yoakim, 440 U.S. 125 (1979).

National Council of Juvenile and Family Court Judges. (1986). *Deprived children: A judicial response.* Reno: University of Nevada.

National Council on Disability. (2000). *Back to school on civil rights.* Washington, DC: U.S. Government Printing Office.

National Institute of Mental Health. (n.d.). *Bipolar disorder.* Retrieved March 30, 2006, from http://www.nimh.nih.gov/healthinformation/bipolarmenu.cfm

Parrish, T., Dubois, J., Delano, C., Dixon, D., Webster, D., Berrick, J. D., & Bolus, S. (2001). *Education of foster group home children, whose responsibility is it? study of the educational placement of children residing in group homes.* Palo Alto, CA: American Institutes of Research.

Pellman, A. (1996). *The ABC's of dependency court.* Los Angeles: Dependency Court Legal Services, Inc., Law Offices of Jo Kaplan.

Pew Commission on Children in Foster Care. (2004). *Fostering the future: Safety, permanence and well-being for children in foster care.* Retrieved May 18, 2004, from http://pewfostercare.org/research/docs/FinalReport.pdf

Pierce v. Society of Sisters, 268 U.S. 510 (1925).

Pollard, J. A., Hawkins, J. D., & Arthur, M. W. (1999). Risk and protection: Are both necessary to understand diverse behavioral outcomes in adolescence? *Social Work Research, 23,* 145-158.

Ramey, C. T. & Ramey, S. L. (2004). Early learning and school readiness: Can early intervention make a difference? *Merrill Palmer Quarterly Journal of Developmental Psychology, 50*(4), 471-491.

Rand Corporation. (March 30, 2005). *Rand study says creating universal preschool in California would create benefits that surpass costs.* Retrieved from: http://www.rand.org/news/press.05/03.30.html.

Rand Corporation. (Spring, 1997). *Preschool year: As the twig is bent.* Retrieved from: http://www.rand.org/publications/randreview/issues/RRR.spring97.children/twig.html.

Reddy, L. & Pfeiffer, S. (1997). Effectiveness of treatment foster are with children and adolescents: A review of outcome studies. *Journal of the American Academy of Child and Adolescent Psychiatry, 36,* 581-588.

Reed, D. F. & Karpilow, K. (2002). *Understanding the child welfare system, in California: A primer for service providers and policymakers.* Berkeley: California Center for Research on Families.

Richardson, W., West, M. A., Day, P., & Stuart, S. (1989). Children with developmental disabilities in the child welfare system: A national survey. *Child Welfare, 68,* 605-612.

Roncker v. Walter 700 F. 2d 1058 (6th Cir. 1983).

Schweitzer, H. & Larsen, J. (2005). *Foster care law: A Primer.* Durham, North Carolina: Carolina Academic Press.

Senate Committee Report on Judiciary Bill No. AB 3553, California (June 23, 1992).

Sibling Placement and Visitation Rights, Md. Code Ann., Fam. Law. §5-525.2 (2006).

Simmel, C. & Price, A. (2002). The shared family care demonstration project: Challenges of implementing and evaluating a community-based project. *Children and Youth Services Review, 24*(6/7), 455-470.

Smithgall, C., Gladden, R. M., Howard, E., George, R., & Courtney, M.E. (2004). *Educational experiences of children in out-of-home care.* Chicago, IL: Chapin Hall Center for Children.

Soler, M. & Shauffer, C. (1990). Fighting fragmentation: Coordination of services for children and families. *Nebraska Law Review, 69,* 278-297.

Special Education Programs (2005). Calif. Educ. Code, Part 30, §56000 et seq.

Swanson, H. L. (1999). Reading research for students with LD: A met-analysis of intervention outcomes. *Journal of Learning Disabilities, 32,* 504-532.

Teichroeb, R. (1999, July 6). Are we failing our foster children? Little being done about their educational needs. *Seattle Post-Intelliger,* p. B1.

Torgesen, J. K. (2005, April). *Effective interventions for older students with reading disabilities: Lessons from research.* Presentation at the annual meeting of the Council for Exceptional Children, Baltimore, MD. Retrieved on March 29, 2007 at http://www.fcrr.org/science/pdf/torgesen/CouncilExceptionalChildren.pdf.

U.S. Department of Education. (2003). *Twenty-fifth annual report to congress on the implementation of the Individuals with Disabilities Education Act.* Washington, DC: U.S. Government Printing Office.

U.S. Department of Health and Human Services Bureau. (1997). *National study of protective, preventive, and reunification services delivered to children and families.* Washington, DC: U.S. Government Printing Office.

U.S. Department of Health and Human Services. (1999). *Title IVE independent living programs: A decade in review.* Washington, DC: U.S. Government Printing Office.

U.S. General Accounting Office. (1995). *Health care needs of many young children are unknown and unmet.* Washington, DC: U.S. Government Printing Office.

Vandivere, S., Chalk, R., & Moore, K. A. (Dec. 2003). *Children in foster homes: How are they faring?* Child Trends Research Brief.#2003-23. Retrieved from: http://www.childtrends.org/files/FosterHomesRB.pdf.

Vaughn, S. R., Moody, S. W., & Shuman, J. S. (1998). Broken promises: Reading instruction in the resource room. *Exceptional Children, 64,* 211-225.

Wagner, M. M. (1995). Outcomes for youths with serious emotional disturbance in secondary school and early adulthood. *The Future of Children, 5*(2), 91-112.

Wald, M. S. & Wolverton, M. (1990). Risk assessment: The emperor's new clothes? *Child Welfare, 69,* 483-511.

Ward, K. M. & Bosek, R. L. (2002). Behavioral risk management: Supporting individuals with developmental disabilities who exhibit inappropriate sexual behaviors. *Research & Practice for Persons with Severe Disabilities, 21*(1), 27-42.

Weatherly, R. & Lipsky, M. (1977). Street-level bureaucrats and institutional innovation: Implementing special-education reform. *Harvard Educational Review, 47,* 171-197.

Weinberg, L. A. (1997). Problems in educating abused and neglected children with disabilities. *Child Abuse and Neglect, 21*(9), 889-906.

Weinberg, L. A. Weinberg, C., & Shea, N. M. (1997). Advocacy's role in identifying dysfunctions in agencies serving abused and neglected children. *Child Maltreatment, 2,* 212-225.

Weinberg, L. A., Zetlin, A. G., & Shea, N. M. (2001). *A review of literature on the educational needs of children involved in family and juvenile court proceedings.* San Francisco CA: Judicial Council of California, Center for Children, Families and the Court.

Weinberg, L. A., Zetlin, A. G., & Shea, N. M. (2004). *The Education Liaison Model.* Los Angeles: Mental Health Advocacy Services, Inc. Retrieved March 12, 2006 at www.mhas-la.org

Weisz, V. G. (1995). *Children and adolescents in need: A legal primer for the helping professional* (p. 27). Thousand Oaks: Sage.

Youth Transition Funders Group. (2004). *Connected by 25: A plan for investing in successful futures for foster youth. Takoma Park, MD: Youth Transition Funders Group.* Retrieved on March 29, 2007 from: http://www.ytfg.org/documents/connectedby25_Foster.pdf. Excerpts reprinted with permission.

Zetlin, A. (2003). Education initiative final report. In L. A. Weinberg, A. G. Zetlin, & N. M. Shea, (Eds.). *The education liaison model.* Los Angeles: Mental Health Advocacy Services, Inc. Retrieved March 11, 2006 at: http://www.mhas-la.org

Zetlin, A. & Weinberg, L. (2004) Understanding the plight of foster youth and improving their educational opportunities. *Child Abuse & Neglect, 28*(9), 917-923.

Zetlin, A., Weinberg, L., & Kimm, C. (2004). Improving education outcomes for children in foster care: Intervention by an education liaison. *Journal of Education for Students Placed At Risk (JESPAR), 9*(4).

Zetlin, A., Weinberg, L. A., & Kimm, C. (2005). Helping social workers address the educational needs of foster children. *Child Abuse & Neglect, 29,* 811-823.

Zetlin, A., Weinberg, L., & Luderer, J. W. (2004). Problems and solutions to improving educational services for children in foster care. *Preventing School Failure, 45*(1), 1-7.

Zetlin, A. G., Weinberg, L. A., & Shea, N. M. (2006a). Seeing the whole picture: Views from diverse participants on barriers to educating foster youth. *Children and Schools, 28*(3), 165-174.

Zetlin, A. G., Weinberg, L. A., & Shea, N. M. (2006b). Improving educational prospects for youth in foster care: The education liaison model. *Intervention in Schools and Clinics, 41*(5), 267-272.

Zetlin, A., Weinberg, L., & Tunick, R. (2002). Advocating to resolve educational problems of children in foster care. *Advisor, 14*(1).

Zima, B. T., Bussing, R., Freeman, S., Yang, X., Belin, T. R., & Forness, S. R. (2000). Behavior problems, academic skill delays and school failure among school-aged children in foster care: Their relationship to placement characteristics. *Journal of Child and Family Studies, 9*(1), 87-103.

Index